This report contains the collective views of an international group of experts and does not necessarily represent the decisions or the stated policy of the United Nations Environment Programme, the International Labour Organisation, or the World Health Organization.

Environmental Health Criteria 127

ACROLEIN

First draft prepared by Dr T. Vermeire,
National Institute of Public Health and
Environmental Protection, Bilthoven, The Netherlands

Published under the joint sponsorship of
the United Nations Environment Programme,
the International Labour Organisation,
and the World Health Organization

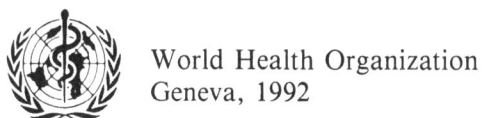

World Health Organization
Geneva, 1992

The **International Programme on Chemical Safety (IPCS)** is a joint venture of the United Nations Environment Programme, the International Labour Organisation, and the World Health Organization. The main objective of the IPCS is to carry out and disseminate evaluations of the effects of chemicals on human health and the quality of the environment. Supporting activities include the development of epidemiological, experimental laboratory, and risk-assessment methods that could produce internationally comparable results, and the development of manpower in the field of toxicology. Other activities carried out by the IPCS include the development of know-how for coping with chemical accidents, coordination of laboratory testing and epidemiological studies, and promotion of research on the mechanisms of the biological action of chemicals.

WHO Library Cataloguing in Publication Data

Acrolein.

(Environmental health criteria ; 127)

1. Acrolein - adverse effects   2. Acrolein - toxicity
3. Environmental exposure   4. Environmental pollutants
I. Series

ISBN 92 4 157127 6   (LC Classification: QD 305.A6)
ISSN 0250-863X

©World Health Organization 1991

Publications of the World Health Organization enjoy copyright protection in accordance with the provisions of Protocol 2 of the Universal Copyright Convention. For rights of reproduction or translation of WHO publications, in part or *in toto*, application should be made to the Office of Publications, World Health Organization, Geneva, Switzerland. The World Health Organization welcomes such applications.

The designations employed and the presentation of the material in this publication do not imply the expression of any opinion whatsoever on the part of the Secretariat of the World Health Organization concerning the legal status of any country, territory, city, or area or of its authorities, or concerning the delimitation of its frontiers or boundaries.

The mention of specific companies or of certain manufacturers' products does not imply that they are endorsed or recommended by the World Health Organization in preference to others of a similar nature that are not mentioned. Errors and omissions excepted, the names of proprietary products are distinguished by initial capital letters.

CONTENTS

ENVIRONMENTAL HEALTH CRITERIA FOR ACROLEIN

1.	SUMMARY	11
2.	IDENTITY, PHYSICAL AND CHEMICAL PROPERTIES, AND ANALYTICAL METHODS	15
	2.1 Identity	15
	2.2 Physical and chemical properties	16
	2.3 Conversion factors	17
	2.4 Analytical methods	17
3.	SOURCES OF HUMAN AND ENVIRONMENTAL EXPOSURE	23
	3.1 Natural sources	23
	3.2 Anthropogenic sources	23
	3.2.1 Production	23
	3.2.1.1 Production levels and processes	23
	3.2.1.2 Emissions	23
	3.2.2 Uses	24
	3.2.3 Waste disposal	24
	3.2.4 Other sources	25
4.	ENVIRONMENTAL TRANSPORT, DISTRIBUTION, AND TRANSFORMATION	27
	4.1 Transport and distribution between media	27
	4.2 Abiotic degradation	27
	4.2.1 Photolysis	28
	4.2.2 Photooxidation	28
	4.2.3 Hydration	30
	4.3 Biotransformation	31
	4.3.1 Biodegration	31
	4.3.2 Bioaccumulation	31
5.	ENVIRONMENTAL LEVELS AND HUMAN EXPOSURE	33
	5.1 Environmental levels	33
	5.1.1 Water	33
	5.1.2 Air	33
	5.2 General population exposure	33
	5.2.1 Air	33

		5.2.2 Food	38
	5.3	Occupational exposure	38
6.	KINETICS AND METABOLISM		40
	6.1	Absorption and distribution	40
	6.2	Reaction with body components	40
		6.2.1 Tracer-binding studies	40
		6.2.2 Adduct formation	41
		6.2.2.1 Interactions with sulfhydryl groups	41
		6.2.2.2 *In vitro* interactions with nucleic acids	42
	6.3	Metabolism and excretion	43
7.	EFFECTS ON LABORATORY MAMMALS AND *IN VITRO* TEST SYSTEMS		46
	7.1	Single exposure	46
		7.1.1 Mortality	46
		7.1.2 Effects on the respiratory tract	46
		7.1.3 Effects on skin and eyes	49
		7.1.4 Systemic effects	49
		7.1.5 Cytotoxicity *in vitro*	50
	7.2	Short-term exposure	53
		7.2.1 Continuous inhalation exposure	53
		7.2.2 Repeated inhalation exposure	54
		7.2.3 Repeated intraperitoneal exposure	58
	7.3	Biochemical effects and mechanisms of toxicity	59
		7.3.1 Protein and non-protein sulfhydryl depletion	59
		7.3.2 Inhibition of macromolecular synthesis	60
		7.3.3 Effects on microsomal oxidation	60
		7.3.4 Other biochemical effects	61
	7.4	Immunotoxicity and host resistance	62
	7.5	Reproductive toxicity, embryotoxicity, and teratogenicity	63
	7.6	Mutagenicity and related end-points	65
		7.6.1 DNA damage	65
		7.6.2 Mutation and chromosomal effects	66
		7.6.3 Cell transformation	69
	7.7	Carcinogenicity	69
		7.7.1 Inhalation exposure	69
		7.7.2 Oral exposure	70
		7.7.3 Skin exposure	71
	7.8	Interacting agents	71

8.	EFFECTS ON HUMANS	73
	8.1 Single exposure	73
	8.1.1 Poisoning incidents	73
	8.1.2 Controlled experiments	74
	8.1.2.1 Vapour exposure	74
	8.1.2.2 Dermal exposure	77
	8.2 Long-term exposure	77
9.	EFFECTS ON OTHER ORGANISMS IN THE LABORATORY AND FIELD	78
	9.1 Aquatic organisms	78
	9.2 Terrestrial organisms	82
	9.2.1 Birds	82
	9.2.2 Plants	82
10.	EVALUATION OF HUMAN HEALTH RISKS AND EFFECTS ON THE ENVIRONMENT	84
	10.1 Evaluation of human health risks	84
	10.1.1 Exposure	84
	10.1.2 Health effects	84
	10.2 Evaluation of effects on the environment	86
11.	FURTHER RESEARCH	88
12.	PREVIOUS EVALUATIONS BY INTERNATIONAL BODIES	89
	REFERENCES	90
	RESUME	112
	RESUMEN	116

WHO TASK GROUP ON ENVIRONMENTAL HEALTH CRITERIA FOR ACROLEIN

Members

Dr G. Damgard-Nielsen, National Institution of Occupational Health, Copenhagen, Denmark

Dr I. Dewhurst, Division of Toxicology and Environmental Health, Department of Health, London, United Kingdom

Dr R. Drew, Toxicology Information Services, Safety Occupational Health and Environmental Protection, ICI Australia, Melbourne, Victoria, Australia

Dr B. Gilbert, Technology Development Company (CODETEC), Cidade Universitaria, Campinas, Brazil (*Rapporteur*)

Dr K. Hemminki, Institute of Occupational Health, Helsinki (*Chairman*)

Dr R. Maronpot, Chemical Pathology Branch, Division of Toxicology, Research and Testing, National Institute of Environmental Health Sciences, Research Triangle Park, North Carolina, USA

Dr M. Noweir, Industrial Engineering Department, College of Engineering, King Abdul Aziz University, Jeddah, Saudi Arabia

Dr M. Wallén, National Chemicals Inspectorate, Solna, Sweden

Secretariat

Ms B. Labarthe, International Register of Potentially Toxic Chemicals, United Nations Environment Programme, Geneva, Switzerland

Dr T. Ng, Office of Occupational Health, World Health Organization, Switzerland

Dr G. Nordberg, International Agency for Research on Cancer, Lyon, France

Professor F. Valić, IPCS Consultant, World Health Organization, Geneva, Switzerland (*Responsible Officer and Secretary*)[a]

Dr T. Vermeire, National Institute of Public Health and Environmental Protection, Bilthoven, The Netherlands

---

[a] Vice-rector, University of Zagreb, Zagreb, Yugoslavia

NOTE TO READERS OF THE CRITERIA DOCUMENTS

Every effort has been made to present information in the criteria documents as accurately as possible without unduly delaying their publication. In the interest of all users of the environmental health criteria documents, readers are kindly requested to communicate any errors that may have occurred to the Manager of the International Programme on Chemical Safety, World Health Organization, Geneva, Switzerland, in order that they may be included in corrigenda.

* * *

A detailed data profile and a legal file can be obtained from the International Register of Potentially Toxic Chemicals, Palais des Nations, 1211 Geneva 10, Switzerland (Telephone No. 7988400 or 7985850).

ENVIRONMENTAL HEALTH CRITERIA FOR ACROLEIN

A WHO Task Group on Environmental Health Criteria for Acrolein met in Geneva from 7 to 11 May 1990. Dr M. Mercier, Manager, IPCS, opened the meeting and welcomed the participants on behalf of the heads of the three IPCS cooperating organizations (UNEP/ILO/WHO). The Task Group reviewed and revised the draft monograph and made an evaluation of the risks for human health and the environment from exposure to acrolein.

The first draft of this monograph was prepared by Dr T. Vermeire, National Institute of Public Health and Environmental Protection, Bilthoven, Netherlands. Professor F. Valić was responsible for the overall scientific content, and Dr P.G. Jenkins, IPCS, for the technical editing.

The efforts of all who helped in the preparation and finalization of the document are gratefully acknowledged.

ABBREVIATIONS

BOD	biochemical oxygen demand
COD	chemical oxygen demand
EEC	European Economic Community
HPLC	high-performance liquid chromatography
LOAEL	lowest-observed-adverse-effect level
NAD	nicotinamide adenine dinucleotide
NADPH	reduced nicotinamide adenine dinucleotide phosphate
NIOSH	National Institute for Occupational Safety and Health (USA)
NOAEL	no-observed-adverse-effect level

1. SUMMARY

Acrolein is a volatile highly flammable liquid with a pungent, choking, disagreeable odour. It is a very reactive compound.

The world production of isolated acrolein was estimated to be 59 000 tonnes in 1975. A still larger amount of acrolein is produced and consumed as an intermediate in the synthesis of acrylic acid and its esters.

Analytical methods are available for the determination of acrolein in various media. The minimum detection limits that have been reported are 0.1 $\mu g/m^3$ air (gas chromatography/mass spectrometry), 0.1 μg/litre water (high-pressure liquid chromatography), 2.8 μg/litre biological media (fluorimetry), 590 $\mu g/kg$ fish (gas chromatography/mass spectrometry), and 1.4 $\mu g/m^3$ exhaust gas (high-pressure liquid chromatography).

Acrolein has been detected in some plant and animal sources including foods and beverages. The substance is primarily used as intermediate in chemical synthesis but also as an aquatic biocide.

Emissions of acrolein may occur at sites of production or use. Important acrolein emissions into the air arise from incomplete combustion or pyrolysis of organic materials such as fuels, synthetic polymers, food, and tobacco. Acrolein may make up 3-10% of total vehicle exhaust aldehydes. Smoking one cigarette yields 3-228 μg acrolein. Acrolein is a product of photochemical oxidation of specific organic air pollutants.

Exposure of the general population will predominantly occur via air. Oral exposure may occur via alcoholic beverages or heated foodstuffs.

Average acrolein levels of up to approximately 15 $\mu g/m^3$ and maximum levels of up to 32 $\mu g/m^3$ have been measured in urban air. Near industries and close to exhaust pipes, levels that are ten to one hundred times higher may occur. Extremely high air levels in the mg/m^3 range can be found as a result of fires. In indoor air, smoking one cigarette per m^3 of room-space in 10-13 min was found to lead to acrolein vapour concentrations of 450-840 $\mu g/m^3$. Workplace levels of over 1000 $\mu g/m^3$ were reported in situations involving the heating of organic materials, e.g., welding or heating of organic materials.

Acrolein is degraded in the atmosphere by reaction with hydroxyl radicals. Atmospheric residence times are about one day.

In surface water, acrolein dissipates in a few days. Acrolein has a low soil adsorption potential. Both aerobic and anaerobic degradation have been reported, although the toxicity of the compound to microorganisms may prevent biodegradation. Based on the physical and chemical properties, bioaccumulation of acrolein would not be expected to occur.

Acrolein is very toxic to aquatic organisms. Acute EC_{50} and LC_{50} values for bacteria, algae, crustacea, and fish are between 0.02 and 2.5 mg/litre, bacteria being the most sensitive species. The 60-day no-observed-adverse-effect level (NOAEL) for fish has been determined to be 0.0114 mg/litre. Effective control of aquatic plants by acrolein has been achieved at dosages of between 4 and 26 mg/litre.h. Adverse effects on crops grown on soil irrigated by acrolein-treated water have been observed at concentrations of 15 mg/litre or more.

In animals and humans the reactivity of acrolein effectively confines the substance to the site of exposure, and pathological findings are also limited to these sites. A retention of 80-85% acrolein was found in the respiratory tract of dogs exposed to 400-600 mg/m^3. Acrolein reacts directly with protein and non-protein sulfhydryl groups and with primary and secondary amines. It may also be metabolized to mercapturic acids, acrylic acid, glycidaldehyde or glyceraldehyde. Evidence for the last three metabolites has only been obtained *in vitro*.

Acrolein is a cytotoxic agent. *In vitro* cytotoxicity has been observed at levels as low as 0.1 mg/litre. The substance is highly toxic to experimental animals and humans following a single exposure via different routes. The vapour is irritating to the eyes and respiratory tract. Liquid acrolein is a corrosive substance. The NOAEL for irritant dermatitis from ethanolic acrolein was found to be 0.1%. Experiments with human volunteers, exposed to acrolein vapour, show a lowest-observed-adverse-effect level (LOAEL) of 0.13 mg/m^3, at which level eyes may become irritated within 5 min. In addition, respiratory tract effects are evident from 0.7 mg/m^3. At higher single exposure levels, degeneration of the respiratory epithelium, inflammatory sequelae, and perturbation of respiratory function develop.

The toxicological effects from continuous inhalation exposure at concentrations from 0.5 to 4.1 mg/m^3 have been studied in rats, dogs, guinea-pigs, and monkeys. Both respiratory tract function and histopathological effects were seen when animals were exposed to acrolein at levels of 0.5 mg/m^3 or more for 90 days.

Summary

The toxicological effects from repeated inhalation exposure to acrolein vapour at concentrations ranging from 0.39 mg/m^3 to 11.2 mg/m^3 have been studied in a variety of laboratory animals. Exposure durations ranged from 5 days to as long as 52 weeks. In general, body weight gain reduction, decrement of pulmonary function, and pathological changes in nose, upper airways, and lungs have been documented in most species exposed to concentrations of 1.6 mg/m^3 or more for 8 h/day. Pathological changes include inflammation, metaplasia, and hyperplasia of the respiratory tract. Significant mortality has been observed following repeated exposures to acrolein vapour at concentrations above 9.07 mg/m^3. In experimental animals acrolein has been shown to deplete tissue glutathione and in *in vitro* studies, to inhibit enzymes by reacting with sulfhydryl groups at active sites. There is limited evidence that acrolein can depress pulmonary host defences in mice and rats.

Acrolein can induce teratogenic and embryotoxic effects if administered directly into the amnion. However, the fact that no effect was found in rabbits injected intravenously with 3 mg/kg suggests that human exposure to acrolein is unlikely to affect the developing embryo.

Acrolein has been shown to interact with nucleic acids *in vitro* and to inhibit their synthesis both *in vitro* and *in vivo*. Without activation it induced gene mutations in bacteria and fungi and caused sister chromatid exchanges in mammalian cells. In all cases these effects occurred within a very narrow dose range governed by the reactivity, volatility, and cytotoxicity of acrolein. A dominant lethal test in mice was negative. The available data show that acrolein is a weak mutagen to some bacteria, fungi, and cultured mammalian cells.

In hamsters that were exposed for 52 weeks to acrolein vapour at a level of 9.2 mg/m^3 for 7 h/day and 5 days/week and were observed for another 29 weeks, no tumours were found. When hamsters were exposed to acrolein vapour similarly for 52 weeks, and, in addition, to intratracheal doses of benzo[*a*]pyrene weekly or to subcutaneous doses of diethylnitrosamine once every three weeks, no clear co-carcinogenic action of acrolein was observed. Oral exposure of rats to acrolein in drinking-water at doses of between 5 and 50 mg/kg body weight per day (5 days/week for 104-124 weeks) did not induce tumours. In view of the limited nature of all these tests, the data for determining the carcinogenicity of acrolein to experimental animals are considered inadequate. In consequence, an evaluation of the carcinogenicity of acrolein to humans is also considered impossible.

The threshold levels of acrolein causing irritation and health effects are 0.07 mg/m^3 for odour perception, 0.13 mg/m^3 for eye irritation, 0.3 mg/m^3 for nasal irritation and eye blinking, and 0.7 mg/m^3 for decreased respiratory rate. As the level of acrolein rarely exceeds 0.03 mg/m^3 in urban air, it is not likely to reach annoyance or harmful levels in normal circumstances.

In view of the high toxicity of acrolein to aquatic organisms, the substance presents a risk to aquatic life at or near sites of industrial discharges, spills, and biocidal use.

2. IDENTITY, PHYSICAL AND CHEMICAL PROPERTIES, AND ANALYTICAL METHODS

2.1 Identity

Chemical formula: C_3H_4O

Chemical structure:

```
            H
            |
     H      C = O
      \    /
       C = C
      /    \
     H      H
```

Relative molecular mass: 56.06

Common name: acrolein

Common synonyms: acraldehyde, acrylaldehyde (IUPAC name), acrylic aldehyde, propenal, prop-2-enal, prop-2-en-1-al

Common trade names: Acquinite, Aqualin, Aqualine, Biocide, Magnicide-H, NSC 8819, Slimicide

CAS chemical name: 2-propenal

CAS registry number: 107-02-8

RTECS registry number: AS 1050000

Specifications: commercial acrolein contains 95.5% or more of the compound and, as main impurities, water (up to 3.0% by weight) and other carbonyl compounds (up to 1.5% by weight), mainly propanal and acetone. Hydroquinone is added as an inhibitor of polymerization (0.1-0.25% by weight) (Hess et al., 1978).

2.2 Physical and chemical properties

Acrolein is a volatile, highly flammable, lacrimatory liquid at ordinary temperature and pressure. Its odour is described as burnt sweet, pungent, choking, and disagreeable (Hess et al., 1978; Hawley, 1981). The compound is highly soluble in water and in organic solvents such as ethanol and diethylether. The extreme reactivity of acrolein can be attributed to the conjugation of a carbonyl group with a vinyl group within its structure. Reactions shown by acrolein include Diels-Alder condensations, dimerization and polymerization, additions to the carbon-carbon double bond, carbonyl additions, oxidation, and reduction. In the absence of an inhibitor, acrolein is subject to highly exothermic polymerization catalysed by light and air at room temperature to an insoluble, cross-linked solid. Highly exothermic polymerization also occurs in the presence of traces of acids or strong bases even when an inhibitor is present. Inhibited acrolein undergoes dimerization above 150 °C. Some physical and chemical data on acrolein are presented in Table 1.

Table 1. Some physical and chemical data on acrolein

Physical state	mobile liquid
Colour	colourless (pure) or yellowish (commercial)
Odour perception threshold	0.07 mg/m^3 [a]
Odour recognition threshold	0.48 mg/m^3 [b]
Melting point	-87 °C
Boiling point (at 101.3 kPa)	52.7 °C
Water solubility (at 20 °C)	206 g/litre
Log n-octanol-water partition coefficient	0.9[c]
Relative density (at 20 °C)	0.8427
Relative vapour density	1.94
Vapour pressure (at 20 °C)	29.3 kPa (220 mmHg)
Flash point (open cup)	-18 °C
Flash point (closed cup)	-26 °C
Flammability limits	2.8-31.0% by volume

[a] Sinkuvene (1970) (see Table 12)
[b] Leonardos et al. (1969) (see Table 12)
[c] Experimentally derived by Veith et al. (1980)

2.3 Conversion factors

At 25 °C and 101.3 kPa (760 mmHg), 1 ppm of acrolein = 2.29 mg/m^3 air and 1 mg of acrolein per m^3 air = 0.44 ppm.

2.4 Analytical methods

A summary of relevant methods of sampling and analysis is presented in Table 2.

Tejada (1986) presented data showing that the air analysis HPLC method employing a 2,4-dinitrophenylhydrazine-coated SP cartridge (Kuwata et al., 1983) is equivalent to that using impingers with 2,4-dinitrophenylhydrazine in acetonitrile (Lipari & Swarin, 1982). The latter method was also evaluated in several laboratories and was found adequate for the evaluation of the working environment (Perez et al., 1984). Nevertheless, the separation of 2,4-dinitrophenylhydrazine derivatives of acrolein and acetone by HPLC can present difficulties (Olson & Swarin, 1985). A highly sensitive electrochemical detection method was found by Jacobs & Kissinger (1982) to be suitable and was later improved by Facchini et al. (1986).

A personal sampling device for firemen, which employs molecular sieves, was described by Treitman et al. (1980). Other sampling methods using solid sorbents coated with 2,4-dinitrophenylhydrazine, as applied by Kuwata et al. (1983) for location monitoring, were found suitable for personal sampling procedures (Andersson et al., 1981; Rietz, 1985).

The NIOSH procedure for industrial air monitoring involves absorption onto N-hydroxymethylpiperazine-coated XAD-2 resin and gas chromatographic analysis of the toluene eluate (US-NIOSH, 1984). This method has been validated by a Shell Development Company analytical laboratory and was not revised by NIOSH in 1989.

Table 2. Sampling, preparation, and analysis of acrolein

Medium	Sampling method	Analytical method	Detection limit	Sample size	Comments	Reference
air	absorption in ethanolic solution of thiosemicarbazide and hydrochloric acid	UV spectrometry	20 µg/m^3	0.02 m^3	suitable for location monitoring; designed for analysis of ambient air; interference from other α, β-unsaturated aldehydes	Manita & Goldberg (1970)
air	absorption in ethanolic solution of 4-hexylresorcinol, mercuric chloride, and trichloroacetic acid	colorimetry	20 µg/m^3	0.05 m^3	suitable for location monitoring; designed for analysis of ambient and industrial air and exhaust gas; slight interference from dienes and α, β-unsaturated aldehydes; also suitable for analysis of smoke	Cohen & Altshuller (1961), Katz (1977), Harke et al. (1972)
air	absorption in aqueous sodium bisulfite; addition of ethanolic solution of 4-hexylresorcinol, mercuric chloride, and trichloroacetic acid; heating	colorimetry	20 µg/m^3	0.06 m^3	suitable for location monitoring; designed for analysis of ambient and industrial air and cigarette smoke	Pfaffli (1982), Katz (1977), Ayer & Yeager (1982)

Table 2 (contd).

Medium	Sampling method	Analytical method	Detection limit	Sample size	Comments	Reference
air	collection on molecular sieve 3A and 13X; desorption by heat; collection in water; reaction with aqueous o-aminobiphenyl-sulfuric acid; heating	fluorimetry	2 $\mu g/m^3$	0.06 m^3	suitable for location monitoring; designed for analysis of ambient air; interference from croton-aldehyde and methylvinyl ketone	Suzuki & Imai (1982)
air	adsorption on Poropak N; desorption by heat	gas chromatography with flame ionization detection	< 600 $\mu g/m^3$	0.003–0.008 m^3	suitable for personal monitoring	Campbell & Moore (1979)
air	adsorption on Tenax GC desorption by heat; cryofocussing	gas chromatography with mass spectrometric detection	0.1 $\mu g/m^3$	0.006–0.019 m^3 (breakthrough volume)	suitable for location and personal monitoring; designed for analysis of ambient air	Krost et al. (1982)
air	cryogradient sampling on siloxane-coated chromosorb W AW; desorption by heat	gas chromatography with flame ionization and mass spectrometric detection	0.1 $\mu g/m^3$	0.003 m^3	suitable for location monitoring; designed for analysis of ambient air	Jonsson & Berg (1983)
air	absorption into ethanol; reaction with aqueous methoxyamine hydrochloride-sodium acetate; bromination; adsorption on SP-cartridge; elution by diethyl ether	gas chromatography with electron capture detection	1 $\mu g/m^3$	0.003–0.04 m^3	suitable for location monitoring; designed for analysis of ambient air	Nishikawa et al. (1986)

Table 2 (contd).

Medium	Sampling method	Analytical method	Detection limit	Sample size	Comments	Reference
air	absorption into aqueous 2,4-DNPH hydrochloride; extraction by chloroform;	gas chromatography with flame ionization detection and anthracene as internal standard	435 $\mu g/m^3$	0.01 m^3	designed for analysis of exhaust gas	Saito et al. (1983)
air	collection in cold trap; warming trap	gas chromatography			designed for analysis of tobacco smoke	Rathkamp et al. (1973)
air	direct introduction	gas chromatography	0.1 g/m^3	2 cm^3	designed for analysis of tobacco smoke	Richter & Erfurnth (1979)
air	adsorption on 2,4-DNPH-phosphoric acid coated SP-cartridge; elution by acetonitrile	HPLC with UV detection	0.5 $\mu g/m^3$	0.1 m^3	suitable for location monitoring; designed for analysis of industrial and ambient air	Kuwata et al. (1983)
air	absorption into solution of 2,4-DNPH-perchloric acid in acetonitrile;	HPLC with UV detection	11 $\mu g/m^3$	0.02 m^3	suitable for location monitoring; designed for analysis of exhaust gas	Lipari & Swarin (1982)
air	absorption into solution of 2-diphenylacetyl-1,3-indandione-1-hydrazone and hydrochloric acid in acetonitrile	HPLC with fluorescence detection	1.4 $\mu g/m^3$	0.02 m^3	suitable for location monitoring; designed for analysis of exhaust gas	Swarin & Lipari (1983)

Table 2 (contd).

Medium	Sampling method	Analytical method	Detection limit	Sample size	Comments	Reference
air	absorption into aqueous 2,4-DNPH-hydrochloric acid and chloroform	HPLC with UV detection	10 µg/cigarette	1 cigarette	designed for analysis of cigarette smoke gas phase	Manning et al. (1983)
air	absorption into 2-(hydroxymethyl) piperidine on XAD-2; elution by toluene	gas chromatography with nitrogen-specific detector	229 µg/m^3	0.05 m^3	suitable for personal monitoring	US-NIOSH (1984)
water	addition of 4-hexyl-resorcinol-mercuric chloride solution and trichloroacetic acid to sample in ethanol	colorimetry	400 µg/litre	0.0025 litre	slight interference from dienes and α, β-unsaturated aldehydes	Cohen & Altshuller (1961)
water	reaction with methoxyl-amine hydrochloride-sodium acetate; bromination; adsorption on SP cartridge; elution by diethyl ether	gas chromatography with electron capture detection	0.4 µg/litre		designed for analysis of rain water	Nishikawa et al. (1987a)
water	reaction with 2,4-DNPH; with addition of iso-octane	HPLC with electro-chemical detection	29 µg/litre		designed for analysis of fog and rain water	Facchini et al. (1986)

Table 2 (contd).

Medium	Sampling method	Analytical method	Detection limit	Sample size	Comments	Reference
water	low pressure distillation; cryofocussing into aqueous 2,4-DNPH-hydrochloric acid; extraction by chloroform; TLC and magnesia-silica-gel column chromatography	HPLC with UV detection	< 0.1 µg/litre	1000 ml	designed for analysis of beer	Greenhoff & Wheeler (1981)
biological media	reaction with aqueous m-aminophenol-hydroxylamine-hydrochloride-hydrochloric acid; heating	fluorimetry	2.8 µg/litre	2 ml	designed for analysis of biological media	Alarcon (1968)
tissue	homogenization; reaction with aqueous 2,4-DNPH-sulfuric acid; extraction by chloroform	HPLC with UV detection				Boor & Ansari (1986)
food	ultrasonic homogenization in cooled water; purging by helium; trapping on Tenax GC-silica-gel-charcoal; desorption by heat	gas chromatography with mass spectrometric detection	590 µg/kg	1000 mg	designed for analysis of volatile organic compounds in fish	Easley et al. (1981)

3. SOURCES OF HUMAN AND ENVIRONMENTAL EXPOSURE

3.1 Natural sources

Acrolein is reported to occur naturally, e.g., in the essential oil extracted from the wood of oak trees (IARC, 1979), in tomatoes (Hayase et al., 1984), and in certain other foods (section 5.2.2.).

3.2 Anthropogenic sources

3.2.1 Production

3.2.1.1 Production levels and processes

In 1975, the worldwide production of acrolein was estimated to be 59 000 tonnes, although at this time production figures probably only related to isolated acrolein (Hess et al., 1978). It is mainly produced in the USA, Japan, France, and Germany. In addition, acrolein is produced as an unisolated intermediate in the synthesis of acrylic acid and its esters. In 1983, 216 000 to 242 000 tonnes of acrolein was reported to be used in the USA for this purpose, amounting to 91-93% of the total production in that country (Beauchamp et al.,1985). Formerly acrolein was produced by vapour phase condensation of acetaldehyde and formaldehyde (Hess et al., 1978). Although this process is now virtually obsolete, some production via this pathway has continued in the USSR (IRPTC, 1984). Worldwide, most acrolein is now produced by the direct catalytic oxidation of propene. Catalysts containing bismuth, molybdenum, and other metal oxides enable a conversion of propene of over 90% and have a high selectivity for acrolein. By-products are acrylic acid, acetic acid, acetaldehyde, and carbon oxides (Hess et al., 1978; Ohara et al., 1987). Another catalyst used for this process, cuprous oxide, has a lower performance (Hess et al., 1978; IRPTC, 1984).

3.2.1.2 Emissions

Closed-systems are used in production facilities, and releases of acrolein to the environment are expected to be low, especially when the compound is directly converted to acrylic acid and its esters. The compound is emitted via exhaust fumes, process waters and waste, and following leakage of equipment. Production losses in the USA in 1978 were estimated to be 35 tonnes or approximately 0.1% of the amount of isolated acrolein produced (Beauchamp et al., 1985).

The air emission factor of acrolein in the synthesis of acrylonitrile in the Netherlands has been reported to be 0.1-0.3 kg per tonne of acrylonitrile (DGEP, 1988). Acrolein has also been identified in the process streams of plants manufacturing acrylic acid (Serth et al., 1978). The application of acrolein as a biocide brings the chemical directly into the aquatic environment.

3.2.2 Uses

The principal use of acrolein is as an intermediate in the synthesis of numerous chemicals, in particular acrylic acid and its lower alkyl esters and DL-methionine, an essential amino acid used as a feed supplement for poultry and cattle. In the USA, in 1983, 91 to 93% of the total quantity of acrolein produced was converted to acrylic acid and its esters, and 5% to methionine (Beauchamp et al., 1985). Other derivatives of acrolein are: 2-hydroxyadipaldehyde, 1,2,6-hexanetriol, lysine, glutaraldehyde, tetrahydro-benzaldehyde, pentanediols, 1,4-butanediol, tetrahydrofuran, pyridine, 3-picoline, allyl alcohol, glycerol, quinoline, homopolymers, and copolymers (Hess et al., 1978).

Among the direct uses of acrolein, its application as a biocide is the most significant one. Acrolein at a concentration of 6-10 mg/litre in water is used as an algicide, molluscicide, and herbicide in recirculating process water systems, irrigation channels, cooling water towers, and water treatment ponds (Hess et al., 1978). About 66 tonnes of acrolein is reported to be used annually in Australia to control submersed plants in about 4000 km of irrigation channels (Bowmer & Sainty, 1977; Bowmer & Smith, 1984). Acrolein protects feed lines for subsurface injection of waste water, liquid hydrocarbon fuels and oil wells against the growth of microorganisms, and at 0.4-0.6 mg/litre it controls slime formation in the paper industry. The substance can also be used as a tissue fixative, warning agent in methyl chloride refrigerants, leather tanning agent, and for the immobilization of enzymes via polymerization, etherification of food starch, and the production of perfumes and colloidal metals (Hess et al., 1978; IARC, 1985).

3.2.3 Waste disposal

Acrolein wastes mainly arise during production and processing of the compound and its derivatives.

Aqueous wastes with low concentrations of acrolein are usually neutralized with sodium hydroxide and fed to a sewage treatment plant for biological secondary treatment. Concentrated wastes are reprocessed whenever possible or burnt in special waste incinerators (IRPTC, 1985).

3.2.4 Other sources

Incomplete combustion and thermal degradation (pyrolysis) of organic substances such as fuels, tobacco, fats, synthetic and natural polymers, and foodstuffs frequently result in the emission of aldehydes. Reported levels are presented in section 5.1.2. Emission rates for several of such sources are presented in Table 3.

The major sources of aldehydes in ambient air formed by incomplete combustion and/or thermal degradation are residential wood burning, burning of coal, oil or natural gas in power plants, burning of fuels in automobiles, and burning of refuse and vegetation (Lipari et al., 1984). Formaldehyde is the major aldehyde emitted, but acrolein may make up 3 to 10 % of total automobile exhaust aldehydes and 1 to 13% of total wood-smoke aldehydes (Fracchia et al., 1967; Oberdorfer, 1971; Lipari et al., 1984). Modern catalytic converters in automobiles almost completely remove these aldehydes from exhaust gases. Acrolein may constitute up to 7% of the aldehydes in cigarette smoke (Rickert et al., 1980).

Aldehydes are also formed by photochemical oxidation of hydrocarbons in the atmosphere. Leach et al. (1964) concluded that formaldehyde and acrolein would constitute 50% and 5%, respectively, of the total aldehyde present in irradiated diluted car exhaust. Acrolein was considered to be mainly a product of oxidation of 1,3-butadiene (Schuck & Renzetti, 1960; Leach et al., 1964), but propene (Graedel et al., 1976; Takeuchi & Ibusuki, 1986), 1,3-pentadiene, 2-methyl-1,3-pentadiene (Altshuller & Bufalini, 1965), and crotonaldehyde (IRPTC, 1984) have also been implicated. The photooxidation of 1,3-butadiene in an irradiated smog chamber, also containing nitrogen monoxide and air, gave rise to the formation of acrolein (55% yield based on 1,3-butadiene initial concentrations). The rate of formation of acrolein was the same as that of 1,3-butadiene consumption. (Maldotti et al., 1980). Cancer chemotherapy patients receiving cyclophosphamide are exposed to acrolein, which results from the metabolism of this drug.

Table 3. Emission rates of aldehydes

Source	Total aldehydes	Formaldehyde	Acrolein	Unit	Reference
Residential wood burning	0.6-2.3	0.089-0.708	0.021-0.132	g/kg	Lipari et al. (1984)
Power plants - coal		0.002		g/kg	Natusch (1978)
- oil		0.1		g/kg	
- natural gas		0.2		g/kg	
Automobiles - petrol	0.01-0.08			g/km	Lipari et al. (1984)
	0.4-2.3	0.2-1.6	0.01-0.16	g/litre	Guicherit & Schulting (1985)
- diesel	8.4-63	4-38		mg/min	Lies et al. (1986)
	0.021		1-2	g/km	Lipari et al. (1984)
	1-2	0.5-1.4	0.03-0.20	g/litre	Guicherit & Schulting (1985)
Vegetation burning				g/litre	Smythe & Karasek (1973)
Cigarette smoking	44	0.0080	0.0002	mg/min	Lies et al. (1986)
	0.003	18	3	g/kg	Lipari et al. (1984)
Pyrolysis of flue-cured tobacco	82-1203		3-228	µg/cigarette	see section 5.2.1
			42-82	µg/g	Baker et al. (1984)
Heating in air (at up to 400 °C) of					
- polyethylene		up to 75	up to 20	g/kg	Morikawa (1976)
- polypropylene		up to 54	up to 8	g/kg	
- cellulose		up to 27	up to 3	g/kg	
- glucose		up to 18	up to 1	g/kg	
- wood		up to 15	up to 1	g/kg	
Smouldering cellulosic materials		0.66-10.02	0.46-1.74	g/kg	
Hot wire cutting (50 cm long at 215 °C) of PVC wrapping film			27-151	ng/cut	Boettner & Ball (1980)

4. ENVIRONMENTAL TRANSPORT, DISTRIBUTION, AND TRANSFORMATION

4.1 Transport and distribution between media

Acrolein is released into the atmosphere during the production of the compound itself and its derivatives, in industrial and non-industrial processes involving incomplete combustion and/or thermal degradation of organic substances, and, indirectly, by photochemical oxidation of hydrocarbons in the atmosphere. Emissions to water and soil occur during production of the compound itself and its derivatives, and through biocidal use, spills, and waste disposal (chapter 3).

Intercompartmental transport of acrolein should be limited in view of its high reactivity, as is discussed in sections 4.2. and 4.3. Considering the high vapour pressure of acrolein, some transfer across the water-air and soil-air boundaries can be expected. In a laboratory experiment Bowmer et al. (1974) explained a difference of 10% between the amount of total aldehydes (acrolein and non-volatile degradation products, see section 4.2) in an open tank and that in closed bottles by volatilization. It was noted that volatilization may be greatly increased by turbulence.

Adsorption to soil, often involving probable reaction with soil components, may impair the transfer of a compound to air or ground water. The tendency of untreated acrolein to adsorb to soil particles can be expressed in terms of K_{oc}, the ratio of the amount of chemical adsorbed (per unit weight of organic carbon) to the concentration of the chemical in solution at equilibrium. Based on the available empirical relationships derived for estimating K_{oc}, a low soil adsorption potential is expected (Lyman et al., 1982). Experimentally, acrolein showed a limited (30% of a 0.1% solution) adsorbability to activated carbon (Giusti et al., 1974).

4.2 Abiotic degradation

Once in the atmosphere, acrolein may photodissociate or react with hydroxyl radicals and ozone. In water, photolysis or hydration may occur. These processes will be discussed in the following sections.

4.2.1 Photolysis

Acrolein shows a moderate absorption of light within the solar spectrum at 315 nm (with a molar extinction coefficient of 26 litre/mol per cm) and therefore would be expected to be photoreactive (Lyman et al., 1982). However, irradiation of an acrolein-air mixture by artificial sunlight did not result in any detectable photolysis (Maldotti et al., 1980). Irradiation of acrolein vapour in high vacuum apparatus at 313 nm and 30-200 °C resulted in the formation of trace amounts of ethene and carbon oxides (Osborne et al., 1962; Coomber & Pitts, 1969).

4.2.2 Photooxidation

Experimentally determined rate constants for the pseudo first order reaction between acrolein and hydroxyl radicals in the atmosphere are presented in Table 4. Also shown are the atmospheric residence times, which can be derived from the rate constants assuming a 12-h daytime average hydroxyl radical concentration of 2×10^{-15} mol/litre (Lyman et al., 1982). The estimated atmospheric residence time of acrolein of approximately 20 h will decrease with increasing hydroxyl radical concentrations in more polluted atmospheres and increase with the decline in temperature, and consequently the rate of reaction, at higher altitudes. Other variations will be caused by seasonal, altitudinal, diurnal, and geographical fluctuations in the hydroxyl radical concentration.

Other potentially significant gas-phase reactions in the atmosphere may occur between acrolein and ozone or nitrate radicals. Experimentally determined rate constants and atmospheric residence times for these reactions are shown in Table 4. The atmospheric residence times were estimated assuming a 24-h average ozone concentration of 1.6×10^{-9} mol/litre (Lyman et al., 1982) and a 12-h night-time average nitrate radical concentration of 4.0×10^{-12} mol/litre (Atkinson et al., 1987). It can be concluded that the tropospheric removal processes for acrolein are dominated by the reaction with hydroxyl radicals. Carbon monoxide, formaldehyde, glycoaldehyde, ketene, and peroxypropenyl nitrate have been identified as products of the reaction between acrolein and hydroxyl radicals (Edney et al., 1982), and glyoxal was also suggested to be one of the reaction products (Edney et al., 1982, 1986b).

Table 4. Rate constants and calculated atmospheric residence times for gas-phase reactions of acrolein.

Reactant	Temperature (°C)	Technique used	Rate constant (litre/mol per sec)	Atmospheric residence time (h)	Reference
OH radical	25	relative rate	16×10^9	17	Maldotti et al. (1980)
	25	relative rate	11.4×10^9	24	Kerr & Sheppard (1981)
	23	absolute rate	20.6×10^9	13	Edney et al. (1982)
	26	relative rate	11.4×10^9	24	Atkinson et al. (1983)
	23	relative rate	12.3×10^9	23	Edney et al. (1986a)
O_3	23	absolute rate	16.9×10^4	1029	Atkinson et al. (1981)
NO_3	25	relative rate	35.5×10^4	391	Atkinson et al. (1987)

As discussed in section 3.2.4, acrolein is also formed by the photochemical degradation of hydrocarbons in general and 1,3-butadiene in particular. When mixtures of acrolein or 1,3-butadiene with nitrogen monoxide and air were irradiated in a smog chamber, the time required for the half-conversion of 1,3-butadiene to acrolein was always shorter than that required for the half conversion of acrolein. It was concluded that in a real atmospheric environment, with continuous emissions of 1,3-butadiene, acrolein will be continuously formed (Bignozzi et al., 1980).

4.2.3 Hydration

Acrolein does not contain hydrolysable groups but it does react with water in a reversible hydration reaction to 3-hydroxypropanal. The equilibrium constant is pH independent and increases appreciably with increasing initial acrolein concentration, presumably because of the reversible dimerization of 3-hydroxypropanal (Hall & Stern, 1950). In more dilute solutions the equilibrium constant was found to approach 12 at 20 °C (Pressman & Lucas, 1942; Hall & Stern, 1950), indicating that approximately 92% of acrolein is in the hydrated form at equilibrium. This agrees well with the equilibrium concentrations found in buffered solutions of acrolein at 21 °C (Bowmer & Higgins, 1976).

The hydration of acrolein is a first order reaction with respect to acrolein. The rate constants are independent of the initial acrolein concentrations but increase with increasing acid concentrations (Pressman & Lucas, 1942; Hall & Stern, 1950) and also when the pH is raised from 5 to 9 (Bowmer & Higgins, 1976). In dilute buffered solutions of acrolein in distilled water the rate constant is 0.015 h^{-1} at 21 °C and pH 7, corresponding to a half-life of 46 h. However, although in laboratory experiments an equilibrium is reached with 8% of the original acrolein and 85% of total aldehydes still present, these do not persist in river waters so that other methods of dissipation must exist (Bowmer et al., 1974; Bowmer & Higgins, 1976; see also section 4.3.1).

The dissipation of acrolein in field experiments in irrigation channels also followed first order kinetics and was faster than could be predicted assuming hydration alone. First order rate constants, based on the data thought to be most reliable varied between 0.104 and 0.208 h^{-1} at pH values of 7.1 to 7.5 and temperatures of 16 to 24 °C. From these rate constants, half-lives of between 3 and 7 h can be calculated (O'Loughlin & Bowmer,

1975; Bowmer & Higgins, 1976; Bowmer & Sainty, 1977). The latter data agree better than the laboratory data with the results of bioassays with bacteria and fish, which show that aged acrolein solutions become biocidally inactive after approximately 120 to 180 h at a pH of 7 (Kissel et al., 1978). Apparently processes other than hydration also contribute to acrolein dissipation, e.g., catalysis other than acid-base catalysis, adsorption, and volatilization (Bowmer & Higgins, 1976).

4.3 Biotransformation

4.3.1 Biodegradation

No biological degradation of acrolein was observed in two BOD_5 tests with unacclimated microorganisms (Stack, 1957; Bridie et al., 1979a) or in an anaerobic digestion test with unacclimated acetate-enriched cultures (Chou et al., 1978). In two of these cases this was explained by the toxicity of the test compound to microorganisms (Stack, 1957; Chou et al., 1978). The BOD_5 of acrolein in river water containing microorganisms acclimated to acrolein over 100 days was found to be 30% of the theoretical oxygen demand (Stack, 1957). Applying methane fermentation in a mixed reactor with a 20-day retention time, seeded by an acetate-enriched culture, a 42% reduction in COD was achieved after 70-90 days of acclimation to a final daily feed concentration of 10 g/litre (Chou et al., 1978). In a static-culture flask-screening procedure, acrolein (at a concentration of 5 or 10 mg/litre medium) was completely degraded aerobically within 7 days, as shown by gas chromatography and by determination of dissolved organic carbon and total organic carbon (Tabak et al., 1981).

As discussed in section 4.2.3, acrolein in water is in equilibrium with its hydration product. Bowmer & Higgins (1976) observed rapid dissipation of this product in irrigation water after a lag period of 100 h at acrolein levels below 2-3 mg/litre and suggested that this could be due to biodegradation.

4.3.2 Bioaccumulation

On the basis of the high water solubility and chemical reactivity of acrolein and its low experimentally determined log n-octanol-water partition coefficient of 0.9 (Veith et al., 1980), no bioaccumulation would be expected. Following the exposure of Bluegill sunfish to ^{14}C-labelled acrolein (13 µg/litre water) for 28 days, the half-time for removal of radiolabel taken up by the fish was more than 7 days (Barrows et al, 1980). Although the accumulation of acrolein derived radioactively in this study was described by the authors as bioaccumulation, it does not represent bioaccumulation of acrolein *per se* but rather incorporation of the radioactive carbon into tissues following the reaction of acrolein with protein sulfhydryl groups or metabolism of absorbed acrolein and incorporation of label into intermediary metabolites (see chapter 6) (Barrows et al., 1980).

5. ENVIRONMENTAL LEVELS AND HUMAN EXPOSURE

5.1 Environmental levels

5.1.1 Water

Concentrations of acrolein measured in various types of water at different locations are summarized in Table 5.

5.1.2 Air

Concentrations of acrolein measured in air at different locations are summarized in Table 6. Sources of acrolein (see chapter 3) are reflected in the levels found.

5.2 General population exposure

5.2.1 Air

The general population can be exposed to acrolein in indoor and outdoor air (Table 6). Levels of up to 32 $\mu g/m^3$ have been measured in outdoor urban air in Japan, Sweden, and the USA. In addition, both smokers and non-smokers are exposed to acrolein as the product of pyrolysis of tobacco. An extensive data base shows a delivery of 3-228 μg of acrolein per cigarette to the smoker via the gas-phase of mainstream smoke, the amount depending on the type of cigarette and smoking conditions (Artho & Koch, 1969; Testa & Joigny, 1972; Rathkamp et al., 1973; Rylander, 1973; Guerin et al., 1974; Hoffmann et al., 1975; Richter & Erfurhrth, 1979; Magin, 1980; Rickert et al., 1980; Manning et al., 1983; Baker et al., 1984). The delivery of total aldehydes was found to be 82-1255 μg per cigarette (Rickert et al., 1980), consisting mainly of acetaldehyde (Harke et al., 1972; Rathkamp et al., 1973). In the mainstream smoke of marijuana cigarettes, 92 μg of acrolein per cigarette was found (Hoffmann et al., 1975). Non-smokers are mainly exposed to the side-stream smoke of tobacco products. Smoking 1 cigarette per m^3 of room-space in 10-13 min was found to lead to acrolein levels in the gas-phase of side-stream smoke of 0.84 mg/m^3 (Jermini et al., 1976), 0.59 mg/m^3 (derived from Harke et al., 1972), and 0.45 mg/m^3 (derived from Hugod et al., 1978). In one of these experiments it was observed that the presence of people in the room reduced the acrolein levels, probably by respiratory uptake

Table 5. Environmental levels of acrolein in water

Type of water	Location	Detection limit (µg/litre)	Levels observed[a] (µg/litre)	Reference
Surface water	USA, irrigation canal, point of application 16 km downstream 32 km downstream 64 km downstream	not reported	100 50 35 30	Bartley & Gangstad (1974)
Ground water	USA, water in community and private wells	0.1-3.0	nd	Krill & Sonzogni (1986)
Fog water	Italy, Po valley	29	nd-120	Facchini et al. (1986)
Rain water	Italy, Po valley	29	nd	Facchini et al. (1986)
Rain water	USA, 4 urban locations USA, 1 urban location	not reported	nd 50[b]	Grosjean & Wright (1983)
Rain water	Japan, source unknown	0.04	nd (2 samples) 1.5-3.1 (3 samples)	Nishikawa et al. (1987a)

[a] nd = not detected
[b] includes acetone

Table 6. Environmental levels of acrolein in air

Type of site	Country	Detection limit ($\mu g/m^3$)	Levels observed[a] (mg/m^3)	Reference
Not defined	The Netherlands		0.001	Guicherit & Schulting (1985)
Urban	Los Angeles, USA	7	nd-0.025	Renzetti & Bryan (1961)
Urban	Los Angeles, USA		0.002-0.032 (average, 0.016)	Altshuller & McPherson (1963)
Urban, busy road	Sweden	0.1	0.012	Jonsson & Berg (1983)
Urban	Japan	0.5	nd	Kuwata et al. (1983)
Urban	Japan	1	0.002-0.004	Nishikawa et al. (1986)
Urban, highway	USSR		nd-0.022	Sinkuvene (1970)
Residential, 100 m from highway	USSR		nd-0.013	Plotnikova (1957)
Industrial, 50 m from petrochemical plant	USSR		2.5 (max. of 25/25 samples)	
2000 m from petrochemical plant			0.64 (max. of 21/27 samples)	
1000 m from oil-seed mill	USSR		0.1-0.2	Chraiber et al. (1964)
150 m from oil-seed mill	USSR		0.32	Zorin (1966)
Near coal coking plant	Czechoslovakia		0.004-0.009 (average, 0.007)	Masek (1972)

Table 6 (contd).

Type of site	Country	Detection limit ($\mu g/m^3$)	Levels observed[a] (mg/m^3)	Reference
Near pitch coking plant	Czechoslovakia		0.101-0.37 (average, 0.223)	Vorob'eva et al. (1982)
Enamelled wire plants (two), 300 m from plants 1000 m from plants "control area"	USSR		0.28-0.36 0.14-0.46 0.001-0.23	
Coffee roasting outlet Incinerator	USA	200 0.5	0.59 0.5-0.6	Levaggi & Feldstein (1970) Kuwata et al. (1983)
Fire-fighters' personal monitors in over 200 structural fires	Boston, USA	1150 (1-litre sample)	> 6.9 (10% of samples) > 0.69 (50% of samples)	Treitman et al. (1980)
Enclosed space of 8 m^3 containing burning household combustibles (15% synthetics)	Japan		> 69 (44% of samples) 1370 (max)	Morikawa & Yanai (1986)
Enclosed space, pyrolysis of 2-5 g of polyethylene foam in 147 litres; chamber at 380 °C chamber at 340 °C chamber at 380 °C, red oak chamber at 245 °C, wax candles chamber combustion of 2-5 g of polyethylene foam	USA		128-355 < 4.6 18.32-412.2 98.47-249.61 4.58-52.67	Potts et al. (1978)
Cooking area, heating of sunflower oil at 160-170 °C	USSR		1.1 (max)	Turuk-Pchelina (1960)

Table 6 (contd).

Type of site	Country	Detection limit ($\mu g/m^3$)	Levels observed[a] (mg/m^3)	Reference
Beside exhaust of cars, unidentified fuel			0.46-27.71	Cohen & Altshuller (1961), Seizinger & Dimitriades (1972), Nishikawa et al. (1986, 1987b)
Beside exhaust of engines, gasoline			0.130-50.6	Sinkuvene (1970), Saito et al. (1983)
diesel			0.58-7.2	Sinkuvene (1970), Klochkovskii et al. (1981), Saito et al. (1983)
Beside exhaust of cars, gasoline			up to 6.1	Hoshika & Takata (1976) Lipari & Swarin (1982)
diesel			0.5-2.1	Smythe & Karasek (1973), Lipari & Swarin (1982), Swarin & Lipari (1983)
ethanol		11	nd	Lipari & Swarin (1982)
Near jet engine			nd-0.12	Miyamoto (1986)

[a] max = maximum; nd = not detected

and condensation onto hair, skin, and clothing, (Hugod et al., 1978). Evidence has also been presented that acrolein is associated with smoke particles. The fraction of acrolein thus associated can be deduced to be 20-75% of the total (Hugod et al., 1978; Ayer & Yeager, 1982).

The 30-min average acrolein levels measured in air grab-samples from four restaurants were between 11 and 23 $\mu g/m^3$, the maximum being 41 $\mu g/m^3$ (Fischer et al., 1978).

5.2.2 Food

In newly prepared beer, acrolein was found at a level of 2 μg/litre in one study (Greenhoff & Wheeler, 1981) but was not detected in another (Bohmann, 1985). Aging can raise the level to 5 μg/litre (Greenhoff & Wheeler, 1981). Higher concentrations were reported in another study (Diaz Marot et al, 1983). However, in this case the eight compounds identified after a single chromatographic procedure, except for acetaldehyde, did not include the principal components identified after three successive chromatographic procedures by the earlier authors (Greenhoff & Wheeler, 1981) so that superimposition of acrolein and other compounds may have occurred.

The identification of acrolein in wines (Sponholz, 1982) followed adjustment of the pH to 8 and distillation procedures that might have generated acrolein from a precursor. Similar restrictions may apply to determinations in brandies (Rosenthaler & Vegezzi, 1955; Postel & Adam, 1983). Heated and aged bone grease contained an average level of 4.2 mg/kg (Maslowska & Bazylak, 1985). Acrolein was further detected as a volatile in "peppery" rums and whiskies (Mills et al., 1954; Lencrerot et al., 1984), apple eau-de-vie (Subden et al., 1986), in white bread (Mulders & Dhont, 1972), cooked potatoes (Tajima et al., 1967), ripe tomatoes (Hayase et al., 1984), vegetable oils (Snyder et al., 1985), raw chicken breast muscle (Grey & Shrimpton, 1966), turkey meat (Hrdlicka & Kuca, 1964), sour salted pork (Cantoni et al., 1969), heated beef fat (Umano & Shibamoto, 1987), cooked horse mackerel (Shimomura et al., 1971), and as a product of the thermal degradation of amino acids (Alarcon, 1976).

5.3 Occupational exposure

Concentrations of acrolein measured at different places of work are summarized in Table 7.

Table 7. Occupational exposure levels

Type of site	Country	Detection limit ($\mu g/m^3$)	Levels observed[a] (mg/m^3)	Reference
Production plant for acrolein and methyl mercaptopropionic aldehyde	USSR		0.1-8.2	Kantemirova (1975, 1977)
Plant manufacturing disposable microscope drapes, polyethylene sheets cut by a hot wire	USA	20	nd-0.07	Schutte (1977)
Workshop where metals, coated with anti-corrosion primers are welded	USSR		0.11-0.57 (venting) 0.73-1.04 (no venting)	Protsenko et al. (1973)
Workshop where metals are gas-cut Workshop where metals (no primer) are welded			0.31-1.04 nd	
Coal-coking plants Pitch-coking plants	Czecho-slovakia		0.002-0.55 0.11-0.493	Masek (1972)
Rubber vulcanization plant	USSR		0.44-1.5	Volkova & Bagdinov (1969)
Expresser and forepress shops in oil seed mills	USSR		2-10[b]	Chraiber et al. (1964)
Plant producing thermoplastics	Finland	20	nd	Pfaffli (1982)
Engine workshops, welding	Denmark	15	0.031-0.605[c]	Rietz (1985)

[a] nd = not detected
[b] It should be noted that these levels exceed normal tolerance.
[c] 3 out of 13 samples

6. KINETICS AND METABOLISM

6.1 Absorption and distribution

The reactivity of acrolein towards free thiol groups (section 6.3) effectively reduces the bioavailability of the substance. Controlled experiments on systemic absorption and kinetics have not been conducted, but there are indications that acrolein is not highly absorbed into the system since toxicological findings are restricted to the site of exposure (see chapters 8 & 9). The fact that McNulty et al. (1984) saw no reduction in liver glutathione following inhalation exposure also suggests that inhaled acrolein does not reach the liver to any great extent (section 7.3.1).

Experiments with mongrel dogs showed a high retention of inhaled acrolein vapour in the respiratory tract. The inhaled vapour concentrations were measured to be between 400 and 600 mg/m^3. Retention was calculated by subtracting the amount recovered in exhaled air from the amount inhaled. The total tract retention at different ventilation rates was 80 to 85%. Upper tract retention, measured after severing the trachea just above the bifurcation, was 72 to 85% and was also independent of the ventilation rate. Lower-tract retention, measured after tracheal cannulation, was 64 to 71% and slightly decreased as ventilation rate increased (Egle, 1972). Evidence for systemic absorption of acrolein from the gastrointestinal tract was reported by Draminski et al. (1983), who identified a low level of acrolein-derived conjugates in the urine of rats after the ingestion of a single dose of 10 mg/kg body weight. This dose killed 50% of the animals in this study.

6.2 Reaction with body components

6.2.1 Tracer-binding studies

The *in vitro* binding of ^{14}C-labelled acrolein to protein has been investigated using rat liver microsomes. Acrolein was found to bind to microsomal protein in the absence of NADPH or in the presence of both NADPH and a mixed-function oxidase inhibitor. Incubation following the addition of free sulfhydryl-containing compounds reduced binding by 70-90%, while the addition of lysine reduced binding by 12%. Using gel electrophoresis-fluorography it was shown that acrolein, incubated with a reconstituted cytochrome P-450 system, migrated mostly with cytochrome P-450. It was concluded that acrolein is capable of alkylating free sulfhydryl groups in cytochrome P-450 (Marinello et al., 1984).

When rats received tritium-labelled acrolein intraperitoneally 24 h after partial hepatectomy, the percentages of total liver radioactivity recovered in the acid-soluble fraction, lipids, proteins, RNA, and DNA were approximately 94, 3.5, 1.2, 0.6, and 0.4%, respectively, during the first 5 h after exposure. Distribution of label was stable for at least 24 h. Acrolein was bound to DNA at a rate of 1 molecule per 40 000 nucleotides.

A similar DNA-binding rate was observed for the green alga *Dunaliella bioculata* at a 10 times higher acrolein concentration (Munsch et al., 1974a). In *in vitro* studies, labelled acrolein was found to bind to native calf thymus DNA and other DNA polymerase templates at rates of 0.5-1 molecule per 1000 nucleotides (Munsch et al., 1974b). In a follow-up experiment with *Dunaliella bioculata*, quantitative autoradiography and electron microscopy showed that the preferential area of cellular fixation for acrolein was the nucleus. This fixation was stable for at least 2 days, while that in the plastid and cytoplasm decreased initially (Marano & Demèstere, 1976). As no adducts were identified in these studies, these data were considered unsuitable for evaluation.

6.2.2 Adduct formation

The findings of the tracer-binding studies (section 6.2.1) are not surprising considering the reactivity of acrolein, which makes the molecule a likely candidate for interactions with protein and non-protein sulfhydryl groups and with primary and secondary amine groups such as occur in proteins and nucleic acids. These reactions are most likely to be initiated by nucleophilic Michael addition to the double bond (Beauchamp et al., 1985; Shapiro et al., 1986). Beauchamp et al. (1985) discussed extensively the interactions with protein sulfhydryl groups and primary and secondary amine groups.

6.2.2.1 Interactions with sulfhydryl groups

The non-enzymatic reaction between equimolar amounts of acrolein and glutathione, cysteine or acetylcysteine in a buffered aqueous solution proceeds rapidly to near-completion, forming stable adducts (Esterbauer et al., 1975; Alarcon, 1976). Acrolein-acetylcysteine and acrolein-cysteine adducts yield on reduction S-(3-hydroxypropyl)mercapturic acid and S-(3-hydroxypropyl)-cysteine, respectively (Alarcon, 1976). The reaction between glutathione and acrolein may be catalysed by glutathione S-transferase, as was shown for acrolein-diethylacetal and crotonaldehyde (Boyland & Chasseaud, 1967). Biochemical and toxicological investigations provide more evidence for the interaction, either enzymatic or non-enzymatic, between acrolein and free sulfhydryl groups. In summary, it has been observed that:

- acrolein exposure of whole organisms or tissue fractions results in glutathione depletion (section 7.3.1);
- co-exposure of organisms to acrolein and free sulfhydryl-containing compounds protects against the biological effects of acrolein (sections 7.3.3, 7.3.4, and 7.5);
- acrolein can inhibit enzymes containing free sulfhydryl groups on their active site (section 7.3);
- glutathione conjugates appear in the urine of acrolein-dosed rats (section 6.3).

6.2.2.2 In vitro interactions with nucleic acids

Non-catalytic reactions occur between acrolein and cytidine monophosphate (Descroix, 1972), deoxyguanosine (Hemminki et al., 1980), and deoxyadenosine (Lutz et al., 1982). Chung et al. (1984) have identified the nucleotides resulting from the reaction between acrolein and deoxyguanosine or calf thymus DNA (at 37 °C and pH 7) in phosphate buffer. The adducts identified were the 6- and 8-hydroxy derivatives of cyclic $1,N^2$-propano-deoxyguanosine. These adducts were shown to be formed in a dose-dependent fashion in Salmonella typhimurium TA100 and TA104 following exposure to acrolein and identification of the DNA adducts by an immunoassay (Foiles et al., 1989; see also section 7.6.2). Shapiro et al. (1986) reported that acrolein reacts with cytosine and adenosine derivatives (at 25 °C and pH 4.2), yielding cyclic $3,N^4$ adducts of cytosine derivatives and $1,N^6$ adducts of adenosine derivatives. The reaction between guanosine and acrolein yields the cyclic $1,N^2$ adduct (at 55 °C and pH 4).

The demonstration that acrolein can cause or enhance the formation of complexes between DNA strands (DNA-DNA crosslinking) and between DNA and cellular proteins (DNA-protein crosslinking) is indirect evidence that acrolein interacts with nucleic acids. This subject is discussed further in section 7.6.1. However, no studies have demonstrated unequivocally the interaction of acrolein with DNA following *in vivo* administration to animals.

6.3 Metabolism and excretion

Acrolein is expected to be eliminated from the body via glutathione conjugation (section 6.2.2.1). Draminski et al. (1983) administered acrolein in corn oil orally to Wistar rats at a dose of 10 mg/kg body weight. The urinary metabolites identified by gas chromatography with mass spectrometric detection were *S*-carboxylethyl-mercapturic acid and its methyl ester, the latter possibly being the result of methylation of the urine samples prior to gas chromatography. In expired air a volatile compound was detected by gas chromatography, which was not identified; it was reported that its retention time did not correspond to that of methyl acrylate, acrolein or allyl alcohol. The reduced form of *S*-carboxylethyl-mercapturic acid, i.e. *S*-hydroxypropyl-mercapturic acid, was identified by paper and gas chromatography as the sole metabolite in the urine of CFE rats injected subcutaneously with a 1% solution of acrolein in arachis oil at a dose of approximately 20 mg/kg body weight (Kaye, 1973). This metabolite was collected within 24 h and accounted for 10.5% of the total dose (uncorrected for a recovery of 58%). These data indicate that conjugation with glutathione may dominate the metabolism of acrolein.

Data obtained *in vitro* show that acrolein can also be a substrate of liver aldehyde dehydrogenase (EC 1.2.1.5) and lung or liver microsomal epoxidase (EC 1.14.14.1) (Patel et al., 1980). Acrolein, at concentrations of approximately 200 mg/litre medium, was oxidized to acrylic acid by rat liver S9 supernatant, cytosol, and microsomes, but not by lung fractions, in the presence of NAD^+ or $NADP^+$. The reaction proceeded faster with NAD^+ as cofactor than with $NADP^+$ and was completely inhibited by disulfiram (Patel et al., 1980). Rikans (1987) studied the kinetics of this reaction: mitochondrial and cytosolic rat liver fractions each contained two aldehyde dehydrogenase activities with K_m values of 22-39 mg/litre and 0.8-1.4 mg/litre. Microsomes contained a high K_m activity. Incubation of rat liver or lung microsomes in the presence of acrolein and NADPH yielded glycidaldehyde and its hydration product glyceraldehyde, showing involvement of microsomal cytochrome P-450-dependent epoxidase (Patel et al., 1980). Postulated pathways of acrolein metabolism are summarized in Figure 1.

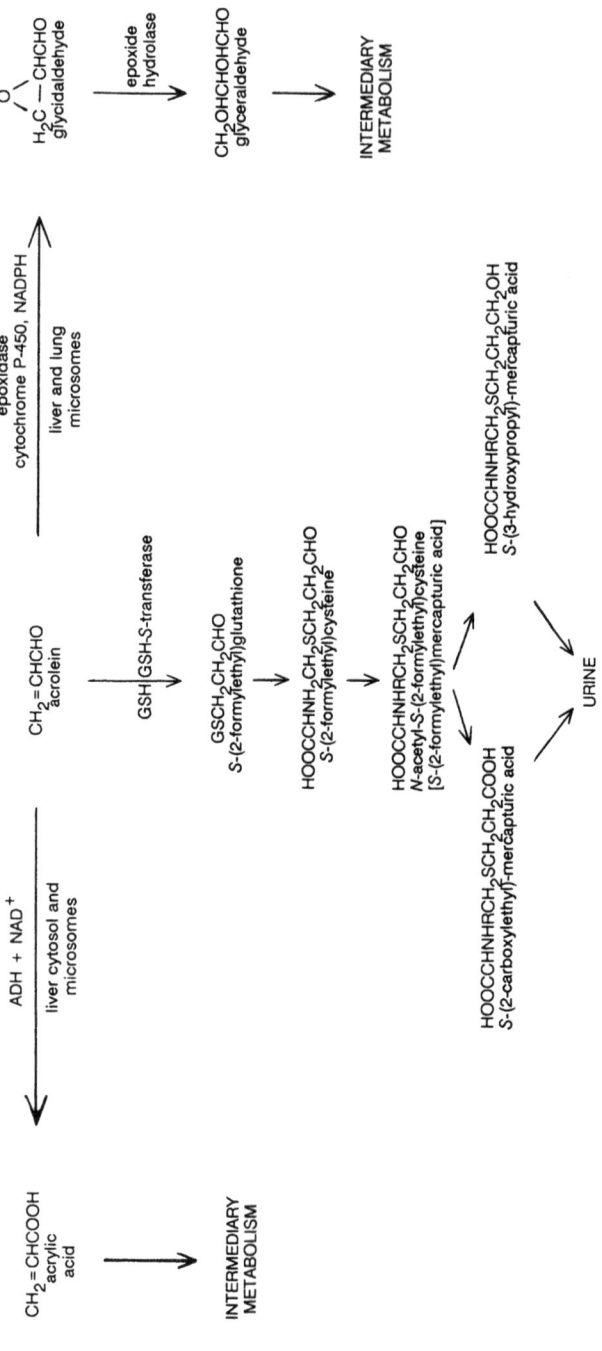

Fig. 1. Proposed metabolism of acrolein
(GSH = glutathione = glutamylcysteinylglycine, ADH = aldehyde dehydrogenase, R=COCH$_3$)

In a human study, the intravenous injection of 1g cyclophosphamide resulted in the excretion of 1.5% acrolein mercapturic acid adduct in the urine (Alarcon, 1976).

As for the fate of the primary metabolites of acrolein, it has been proposed that acrylic acid is methylated and subsequently conjugated to yield S-carboxyl-ethylmercapturic acid, which is a known metabolite of methyl acrylate (Draminski et al., 1983). However, methyl acrylate has never been reported as a metabolite of either acrolein or acrylic acid. It seems more likely that acrylic acid is incorporated into normal cellular metabolism via the propionate degradative pathway (Kutzman et al., 1982; Debethizy et al., 1987). Glycidaldehyde has been shown to be a substrate for lung and liver cytosolic glutathione S-transferase (EC 2.5.1.18) and can also be hydrated to glyceraldehyde (Patel et al., 1980). Glyceraldehyde can be metabolized via the glycolytic pathways.

7. EFFECTS ON LABORATORY MAMMALS AND *IN VITRO* TEST SYSTEMS

7.1 Single exposure

7.1.1 Mortality

The available acute mortality data are summarized in Table 8. Most tests for the determination of the acute toxicity of acrolein do not comply with present standards. Nevertheless, retesting is not justified for ethical reasons and in view of the overt high toxicity of acrolein following inhalation or oral exposure (Hodge & Sterner, 1943).

In addition to the data in Table 8, an oral LD_{95} of 11.2 mg/kg body weight for Charles River rats, observed for 24 h, has been reported (Sprince et al., 1979). Draminski et al. (1983) reported the deaths of 5/10 rats given 10 mg/kg body weight in corn oil by gavage.

7.1.2 Effects on the respiratory tract

In vapour exposure tests, the effects observed in experimental animals have almost exclusively been local effects on the respiratory tract and eyes.

In the LC_{50} studies, effects on the respiratory tract were clinically observed as nasal irritation and respiratory distress in rats (Skog, 1950; Potts et al., 1978; Crane et al., 1986), hamsters (Kruysse, 1971), mice, guinea-pigs, and rabbits (Salem & Cullumbine, 1960) at exposure levels of between 25 mg/m^3 for 4 h and 95 150 mg/m^3 for 3 min. Rats exposed for 10 min to concentrations of 750 or 1000 mg/m^3 suffered asphyxiation (Catilina et al., 1966).

Histopathological investigations in experiments with vapour-exposed rats (Skog, 1950; Catilina et al., 1966; Potts et al., 1978; Ballantyne et al., 1989), hamsters (Kilburn & McKenzie, 1978), guinea-pigs (Dahlgren et al., 1972; Jousserandot et al, 1981), and rabbits (Beeley et al., 1986) revealed varying degrees of degeneration of the respiratory epithelium consisting of deciliation (see also *in vitro* work on cytotoxicity discussed in 7.1.5), exfoliation, necrosis, mucus secretion, and vacuolization. Also observed were acute inflammatory changes consisting of

Table 8. Acute mortality caused by acrolein

Species/strain	Sex	Route of exposure	Observation period (days)	LD (mg/kg bw) or LC$_{50}$ (mg/m^3)[a]	Reference
Rat (Wistar)	male	inhalation (10 min)	8	750	Catilina et al. (1966)[b]
Rat (Wistar)	not reported	oral	14	46 (39-56)	Smyth et al. (1951)[g]
Rat (unspecified strain)	not reported	inhalation (30 min)	21	300	Skog (1950)[b,c]
Rat (Sprague-Dawley)	male	inhalation (30 min)	14	95-217	Potts et al. (1978)[d]
Rat (Sprague-Dawley)	male and female	inhalation (1 h) inhalation (4 h)	14 14	65 (60-68) 20.8 (17.5-24.8)	Ballantyne et al. (1989)
Rat (Sherman)	male and female	inhalation (4 h)	14	18	Carpenter et al. (1949)[b,e]
Hamster (Syrian golden)	male and female	inhalation (4 h)	14	58 (54-62)	Kruysse (1971)
Mouse (unspecified strain)	male	inhalation (6 h)	1	151	Philippin et al. (1970)[f]
Mouse (NMRI)	not reported	intraperitoneal	6	7	Warholm et al. (1984)[g]

[a] Where available, 95% confidence limits are given in parentheses.
[b] Determination of acrolein levels was not reported.
[c] No mortality at 100 mg/m^3, 100% mortality at 700 mg/m^3.
[d] Approximate value: no mortality at 33 mg/m^3, 1/7 and 7/7 died at 95 and 217 mg/m^3, respectively.
[e] Approximate value: 2-4/6 died.
[f] No mortality at 71 mg/m^3, 100% mortality at 273 mg/m^3.
[g] The vehicle was water.

infiltration of white blood cells into the mucosa, hyperaemia, haemorrhages, and intercellular oedema. Proliferative changes of the respiratory epithelium, in the form of early stratification and hyperplasia, were observed in hamsters 96 h after exposure to 13.7 mg/m^3 for 4 h (Kilburn & McKenzie, 1978).

Functional changes in the respiratory system following acrolein vapour exposure have been investigated in guinea-pigs and mice. A rapidly reversible increase in respiratory rate was observed in intact guinea-pigs during exposure to 39 mg/m^3 for 60 min (Davis et al., 1967) and to 0.8 mg/m^3 or more for 2 h (Murphy et al., 1963) followed by a decrease in respiratory rate and an increase in tidal volume. No changes in pulmonary compliance were reported. Davis et al. (1967) did not observe these effects in tracheotomized animals and concluded that they were caused by reflex stimulation of upper airway receptors and not by bronchoconstriction. Murphy et al. (1963), observing that anticholinergic bronchodilators, aminophylline and isoproterenol, but not antihistaminics, reduced the acrolein-induced increase in respiratory resistance, concluded that acrolein caused bronchoconstriction mediated through reflex cholinergic stimulation. In another experiment, an increase in respiratory resistance was also observed in anaesthetized, tracheotomized guinea-pigs with transected medulla during exposure to 43 mg/m^3 for up to 5 min (Guillerm et al., 1967b). The effect was not reversed by atropine. It was concluded by the authors that acrolein did not cause bronchoconstriction via reflex stimulation, but probably via histamine release. When anaesthetized mice were exposed to 300 or 600 mg/m^3 for 5 min via a tracheal cannula, respiratory resistance, respiratory rate, and tidal volume decreased and pulmonary compliance increased at an unspecified time after exposure (Watanabe & Aviado, 1974).

The concentration that produces a 50% decrease in respiratory rate (RD_{50}) as a result of reflex stimulation of trigeminal nerve endings in the nasal mucosa (sensory irritation) has been used as an index of upper respiratory tract irritation. This effect reduces the penetration of noxious chemicals into the lower respiratory tract. The rate of respiration was measured in a body plethysmograph, only the animals' heads being exposed to the acrolein vapour. Depending on the strain, RD_{50} values for mice ranged from 2.4 to 6.6 mg/m^3 (Kane & Alarie, 1977; Nielsen et al., 1984; Steinhagen & Barrow, 1984). In rats a RD_{50} of 13.7 mg/m^3 was found (Babiuk et al., 1985).

7.1.3 Effects on skin and eyes

Animal skin irritation tests have not been performed and skin irritation has not been mentioned as an effect in the acute inhalation tests reported.

One special *in vivo* eye irritation test involved vapour-exposed and control rabbits. At analysed concentrations of acrolein (method not specified) between 4.3 and 5.9 mg/m^3, maintained over 4 h, slight chemosis was observed but no iritis (Mettier et al., 1960). Eye irritation was observed clinically in rodents in several acute inhalation tests, but was not graded (Skog, 1950; Salem & Cullumbine, 1960; Kruysse, 1971; Potts et al., 1978).

7.1.4 Systemic effects

With respect to systemic effects, most studies have been performed at concentrations far above the lethal dose. When rats were exposed to concentrations of acrolein between 1214 and 95 150 mg/m^3 during various periods of time, incapacitation, indicated by the inability to walk in a rotating cage, and convulsions were observed after 2.8 min at the highest concentration and after 27 to 34 min at the lowest concentration. These effects were followed by death after several minutes. Cyanosis of the extremities and agitation were observed at levels of 22 900 mg/m^3 or more (Crane et al., 1986).

The effects of acrolein on the cardiovascular system were investigated by Egle & Hudgins (1974). Rats anaesthetized by sodium pentobarbital and exposed only via the mouth and nose to concentrations between 10 and 5000 mg/m^3 for 1 min showed an increase in blood pressure at all exposure levels. The heart rate was increased at concentrations from 50 mg/m^3 to 500 mg/m^3 but decreased at 2500 and 5000 mg/m^3. Intravenous experiments suggested that increased blood pressor responses resulted from the release of catecholamines from sympathetic nerve endings and from the adrenal medulla and that the decreased heart rate effect was mediated by the vagus nerve (Egle & Hudgins, 1974).

In an acute oral test with rats exposed at 11.2 mg/kg body weight, decreased reflexes, body sag, poor body tone, lethargy, stupor, and tremors were observed, as well as respiratory distress (Sprince et al., 1979).

Because acrolein was shown to induce acute cytotoxicity of the rat urinary bladder mucosa when instilled directly into the bladder lumen (Chaviano et al., 1985), this end-point was investigated *in vivo*. Two days after a single oral or intraperitoneal dose of 25 mg/kg body weight to ten rats per group, focal simple hyperplasia of the urinary bladder was detected in the three surviving rats dosed intraperitoneally. None of the orally exposed rats showed this effect, but all exhibited severe erosive haemorrhagic gastritis. Both orally and intraperitoneally exposed rats showed eosinophilic degeneration of hepatocytes. No abnormalities were observed in sections of lungs, kidneys, and spleen. Acrolein was also administered intraperitoneally at single doses of 0.5, 1, 2, 4, or 6 mg/kg body weight. Proliferation of the bladder mucosa was evaluated autoradiographically by measuring [^{3}H-methyl]thymidine incorporation in exposed versus control rats 5 days after the intraperitoneal injection of acrolein and was found to be increased nearly two-fold at the highest dose. Body weight gain was decreased at the two highest doses. Histopathological evaluation of the liver and urinary bladder did not reveal abnormalities (Sakata et al., 1989).

7.1.5 Cytotoxicity in vitro

As shown in Table 9, mammalian cell viability is affected by acrolein *in vitro* at nominal concentrations of 0.1 mg/litre or more (not corrected for interaction with culture medium components or volatilization). The concentration at which formaldehyde exhibited a similar degree of cytotoxicity was about 6 to 100 times higher (Holmberg & Malmfors, 1974; Pilotti et al., 1975; Koerker et al., 1976; Krokan et al., 1985).

Acrolein is a known inhibitor of respiratory tract ciliary movement *in vitro*. After a 20-min exposure to an acrolein concentration of 34-46 mg/m^3, the ciliary beating frequency of excised sheep trachea decreased by 30% (Guillerm et al., 1967a). Exposure to 13 mg/m^3 for 1 h is the greatest exposure that does not stop ciliary activity in excised rabbit trachea (Dalhamn & Rosengren, 1971). The no-observed-effect-level for longer exposure periods would be expected to be lower than 13 mg/m^3. Other *in vitro* investigations into the inhibition of ciliary movement by acrolein were reviewed by Izard & Libermann (1978).

Table 9. *In vitro* cytotoxicity of acrolein

Cell type	Exposure period (h)	Effect	Concentration (mg/litre medium)	Reference
Rat cardiac fibroblasts/myocytes	4	increased lactate dehydrogenase release	≥ 2.8	Toraason et al. (1989)
Rat cardiac myocytes	2	abolished myocine beat dehydrogenase	≥ 2.8	
	4	decreased ATP levels	≥ 0.56	
Mouse Ehrlich Landschutz	5	92% survival[a]	1	Holmberg & Malmfors (1974)
Diploid ascites tumour cells	5	53% survival[a]	5	
Mouse B P8 ascites sarcoma cells	48	20% growth rate inhibition	0.6	Pilotti et al. (1975)
	48	94% growth rate inhibition	5.6	
Mouse C1300 neuroblastoma cells	24	50% survival[a]	1.7	Koerker et al. (1976)
Mouse L 1210 leukaemia cells	1	70-80% survival[a]	1.1	Wrabetz et al. (1980)
	1	< 15% survival[a]	2.8	
Chinese hamster ovary cells	5	100% mitotis inhibition	0.6	Au et al. (1980)
Adult human bronchial fibroblasts	1	92% colony-forming efficiency	0.06	Krokan et al. (1985)
	1	45% colony-forming efficiency	0.2	

Table 9 (contd).

Cell type	Exposure period (h)	Effect	Concentration (mg/litre medium)	Reference
Adult human lymphocytes	48	decreased replicative index	0.6	Wilmer et al. (1986)
	48	100% mitosis inhibition	2.2	
Human K562 chromic myeloid leukaemia cells	1	marked reduction in colony-forming ability	> 0.3	Crook et al. (1986a,b)
Human bronchial epithelial cells	1	20% colony-forming efficiency	0.06	Grafström et al. (1988)
	1	50% colony-forming efficiency	0.06–0.17	
	1	50% survival[a]	0.34	
	3	clonal growth rate inhibition	≥ 0.17	
	3	increase in cross-linkage envelope formation	≥ 0.06	
	3	decreased plasminogen activator activity	≥ 0.56	
Human fibroblasts	5	63% cell count reduction	< 0.017	Curren et al. (1988)
DNA-repair deficient human fibroblasts	5	63% cell count reduction	0.045	

[a] measured as dye exclusion

7.2 Short-term exposure

7.2.1 Continuous inhalation exposure

In two subchronic inhalation studies with rats, changes in weight gain, longevity, behaviour, and several physiological parameters were reported (Gusev et al., 1966; Sinkuvene, 1970). Unfortunately, the reports did not give sufficient details on the exposure conditions and protocols and the studies are thus of limited value in evaluating the toxicological properties of acrolein.

Groups of 7 or 8 Sprague-Dawley rats of both sexes, 7 or 8 Princeton or Hartley-derived guinea-pigs of both sexes, 2 male pure-bred Beagle dogs, and 9 male squirrel-monkeys were exposed to a vapourized acrolein-ethanol-water mixture for 90 days (Lyon et al., 1970). The measured acrolein concentrations were 0, 0.5 (two groups for each species), 2.3, and 4.1 mg/m^3 and the ethanol concentrations were below 18.7 mg/m^3. Pathological investigations did not include weighing of tissues and organs or examination of the tracheas at the lowest exposure level. There was no treatment-related mortality. One monkey died at 0.5 mg/m^3 and one at 2.3 mg/m^3 due to accidental infections. Body weight gain reduction was only found in rats at 2.3 and 4.1 mg/m^3. Clinically, ocular discharge and salivation were observed in dogs at 2.3 and 4.1 mg/m^3 and in monkeys at 4.1 mg/m^3. Monkeys kept their eyes closed at 2.3 mg/m^3. No adverse effects on haematological or biochemical parameters were observed in any of the animals. At necropsy, occasional pulmonary haemorrhage and focal necrosis in the liver were found in three rats at 2.3 mg/m^3. Pulmonary inflammation and occasional focal liver necrosis were also observed in guinea-pigs at this concentration. Sections of lung from two of the four dogs exposed at 0.5 mg/m^3 revealed focal vacuolization, hyperaemia, and increased secretion of bronchiolar epithelial cells, slight bronchoconstriction, and moderate emphysema. At 2.3 mg/m^3, focal inflammatory reactions involved lung, kidney, and liver. Bronchiolitis and early broncho-pneumonia were seen in one dog. At 4.1 mg/m^3, both dogs had confluent bronchopneumonia. All nine monkeys at 4.1 mg/m^3 showed squamous metaplasia and six of them showed basal cell hyperplasia in the trachea. None of the species revealed other treatment-related changes (Lyon et al., 1970).

Bouley et al. (1975) exposed a total of 173 male SPF-OFA rats to a measured acrolein vapour concentration of 1.26 mg/m^3 for a period of 15 to 180 days and used control groups of equal size. No mortality occurred. Sneezing was observed from day 7 to day 21 in the treated animals, and body weight gain and food consumption were reduced. There was an increase in relative lung weight in rats killed on day 77 but not in rats killed on days 15 or 32. The relative liver weight was decreased at day 15 but not thereafter, and the number of alveolar macrophages was decreased at days 10 and 26 but not at days 60 or 180. When groups of 16 rats were infected by one LD_{50} dose of airborne *Salmonella enteriditis* on day 18 or day 63, mortality increased from 53% in controls to 94% in the exposed rats infected on day 18. No changes were observed in biochemical parameters, including the amount of liver DNA per mg of protein in a group of partially hepatectomized rats, or in the response of spleen lymphocytes to phytohaemagglutinin in rats exposed for 39 to 57 days. Other end-points were not investigated.

7.2.2 Repeated inhalation exposure

Lyon et al. (1970) exposed groups of rats, guinea-pigs, dogs, and monkeys to acrolein vapour at concentrations of 0, 1.6. and 8.5 mg/m^3 for 8 h per day and 5 days per week over 6 weeks. With the exception of the exposure levels, period, and frequency, the protocol was the same as that for the continuous inhalation exposure described in section 7.2.1. Two deaths occurred among the nine monkeys at 8.5 mg/m^3. There was body weight gain reduction in rats and body weight loss (not statistically significant) in monkeys at 8.5 mg/m^3. Clinically, eye irritation and salivation were observed in dogs and monkeys and difficult breathing in dogs at 8.5 mg/m^3. No adverse effects on haematological or biochemical parameters were observed in any of the animals. At necropsy, sections of lung from all animals exposed to 1.6 mg/m^3 showed chronic inflammatory changes. Additionally, some showed emphysema. At 8.5 mg/m^3, squamous metaplasia and basal cell hyperplasia were observed in the trachea of both dogs and monkeys. In addition, bronchopneumonia was noted in dogs and necrotizing bronchitis and bronchiolitis in monkeys. Focal calcification of the tubular epithelium was noted in the kidneys of rats and monkeys at 8.5 mg/m^3.

Groups of male Sprague-Dawley rats were also exposed to acrolein vapour at measured concentrations of 0, 0.39, 2.45, and 6.82 mg/m^3 for 6 h per day and 5 days per week over 3 weeks (Leach et al., 1987). Subgroups were used for immunological investigations (section 7.4) and for histopathological examination of nasal turbinates and lungs. Body weight gain was depressed from week 1 up to the end of the exposure period at 6.82 mg/m^3.

Absolute, but not relative, spleen weight was reduced at this exposure level. There were no histological effects on the lungs, but the respiratory epithelium of the nasal turbinates showed exfoliation, erosion, and necrosis, as well as dysplasia and squamous metaplasia at 6.82 mg/m^3. In addition, the mucous membrane covering the septum and lining the floor of the cavity showed hyperplasia and dysplasia (Leach et al., 1987).

Another experiment involved Dahl rats of two lines, one susceptible (DS) and one resistant (DR) to salt-induced hypertension (Kutzman et al., 1984). Groups of 10 female rats of each line were exposed to measured acrolein concentrations of 0, 0.89, 3.21, and 9.07 mg/m^3 for 6 h per day and 5 days per week over 61-63 days. One week after the exposure, survivors were killed for pathological and compositional analysis of the lung following behavioural and clinical chemistry testing. At 9.07 mg/m^3, all DS rats died within 11 days and 4 DR rats died within the exposure period. Reduced body weights were measured in the surviving DR rats during the first 3 weeks, followed by an almost normal body weight gain. Biochemical changes were found in DR rats at 9.07 mg/m^3 and included increases in lung hydroxyproline and elastin, serum phosphorus, and in the activities of serum alkaline phosphatase, alanine aminotransferase (EC 2.6.1.2), and aspartate aminotransferase (EC 2.6.1.1). No effects were observed on exploratory behaviour, locomotor activity, blood pressure, lung protein, blood urea nitrogen, or on serum creatinine, uric acid, or calcium. At necropsy of survivors, DR rats exposed to 9.07 mg/m^3 had increased relative weights of several organs, especially the lungs. It was noted by the authors that the exposed rats gained a considerable amount of weight during the week following exposure. In both rat lines, concentration-related increases were observed in lymphoid aggregates in pulmonary parenchyma, in collections of intra-alveolar macrophages with foamy cytoplasm, and in hyperplastic/metaplastic terminal bronchiolar epithelial changes. Multifocal interstitial pneumonitis and squamous metaplasia of the tracheal epithelium were also found in DR rats exposed to 9.07 mg/m^3. In contrast, dead and moribund rats, especially those of the DS strain, mainly exhibited severe bronchial and bronchiolar epithelial necrosis with exfoliation, oedema, haemorrhage, and varying degrees of bronchopneumonia. Adverse effects were absent in nasal turbinates and in non-pulmonary tissues (Kutzman et al., 1984).

In follow-up studies, groups of 32 to 57 male Fischer-344 rats were exposed in exactly the same way as described for the Dahl rats. Surviving rats were tested for pulmonary function one week after exposure and then killed and examined for compositional analysis, morphometry, and (in nine rats per group) pathological changes in the lung (Kutzman et al., 1985; Costa et al., 1986). At 9.07 mg/m^3, 56% mortality occurred. After an initial body weight loss over the first 10 days, weight gain became comparable to that of controls. There was an increase in the relative weight of several organs, especially the lungs. Lungs also showed an increase in water content and in the levels of elastin and hydroxyproline, but not in the levels of protein and DNA. The hydroxyproline level was also elevated at 3.21 mg/m^3. Histologically, surviving rats treated with 3.21 or 9.07 mg/m^3 demonstrated an exposure-related increase in effects on the respiratory tract consisting of bronchiolar epithelial necrosis with exfoliation, bronchiolar mucopurulent plugs, an increase in bronchiolar and alveolar macrophages, and focal pneumonitis. At 3.21 mg/m^3, there was type II cell hyperplasia and at 9.07 mg/m^3 tracheal, peribronchial, and alveolar oedema and acute rhinitis. The severity of lung lesions was highly variable and three of the nine rats examined at 9.07 mg/m^3 did not exhibit histological damage. Moribund rats mainly showed severe acute bronchopneumonia and focal alveolar and tracheal oedema with exfoliation in the bronchi and bronchioles (Kutzman et al., 1985). In another report from the same research group, the results of pulmonary function testing and morphometry disclosed air-flow dysfunction at 9.07 mg/m^3, which was correlated with the presence of focal peribronchial lesions and the lung elastin concentrations. In contrast, the rats exposed at 0.89 mg/m^3 exhibited enhanced flow-volume dynamics, whereas no effects on lung function were present in the 3.21-mg/m^3 group (Costa et al., 1986).

Groups of six Wistar rats and ten Syrian golden hamsters of both sexes were exposed to acrolein vapour at measured concentrations of 0, 0.9, 3.2, and 11.2 mg/m^3 for 6 h per day and 5 days per week over 13 weeks (Feron et al., 1978). Within the first month of exposure to 11.2 mg/m^3, half the number of rats of each sex died. One hamster died at this exposure level because of renal failure. A treatment-related decrease in body weight gain and food intake was observed in rats exposed to 3.2 mg/m^3 or more. Hamsters showed decreased body weight gain at 11.2 mg/m^3, but food intake was not examined. At this exposure level, all animals kept their eyes closed, rats showed bristling hair, and hamsters showed salivation and nasal discharge. Haematological investigation and urinalysis in week 12 showed no changes in rats. In hamsters, urinalysis revealed no changes, but females showed increases in the number of erythrocytes, packed cell volume, haemoglobin content, and number of lymphocytes and a decrease in the number of neutrophilic leucocytes. Changes in relative organ weights, which were considered by the authors to be related to the treatment, were found in the lung, heart, and kidneys of both species and in the adrenals of rats exposed to 11.2 mg/m^3. Histological changes were confined to the respiratory tract. In the nose, rats exhibited an exposure-related increase in squamous metaplasia and neutrophilic infiltration of the mucosa at levels of 0.9 mg/m^3 or more (at 0.9 mg/m^3 each effect was observed in one male) and occasional necrotizing rhinitis at 11.2 mg/m^3. Hamsters also showed these effects at 11.2 mg/m^3 but only minimal inflammatory changes at 3.2 mg/m^3. In the larynx and trachea of rats exposed to 11.2 mg/m^3, squamous metaplasia was also observed and was accompanied by hyperplasia in bronchi and bronchioli. At this exposure level, the larynx of hamsters was slightly thickened and focal hyperplasia and metaplasia were found in the trachea. Inflammatory changes were present in the bronchi, bronchioli, and alveoli of rats and included haemorrhage, oedema, accumulations of alveolar macrophages, an increase in mucus-producing cells in the bronchioli, and bronchopneumonia. The authors noted considerable variation between individual rats in the degree of the lesions (Feron et al., 1978).

Feron & Kruysse (1977) exposed groups of 36 Syrian golden hamsters of both sexes to acrolein vapour at measured levels of 0 and 9.2 mg/m^3 for 7 h per day and 5 days per week over 52 weeks. Except for 6 males and 6 females, the hamsters were observed for a further 29 weeks after the exposure period. Overall mortality was 38% in exposed hamsters and 33% in controls. Body weight was slightly and reversibly decreased at the end of the exposure period. The other effects observed at the end of the exposure period were essentially similar (but less severe) to those described above for hamsters exposed to 11.2 mg/m^3 for 13 weeks, but hyperplasia was not observed. Histological changes were restricted to the anterior half of the nasomaxillary turbinates and were still found in 20% of the animals at week 81. At that time they mainly consisted of a thickened submucosa and exudation into the lumen. Epithelial metaplasia, but not hyperplasia, was noted. No tumours were found.

Histopathological examination of the respiratory tract of male Swiss-Webster mice was the object of a study involving groups of 16 to 24 male mice exposed to measured concentrations of 3.9 mg/m^3 for 6 h per day during 5 days (Buckley et al., 1984). The lesions observed were restricted to the nose and were most severe in the anterior respiratory epithelium and on the free margins of the nasomaxillary turbinates and the adjacent nasal septum. They consisted of severe deciliation, moderate exfoliation, erosion, ulceration and necrosis, severe squamous metaplasia, moderate neutrophilic infiltration, and a slight serofibrinous exudate. Lesions in the olfactory epithelium were largely confined to the dorsal meatus and consisted of moderate ulceration and necrosis, and slight squamous metaplasia. The nasal squamous epithelium was not affected (Buckley et al., 1984).

One special investigation concerned the effects of acrolein vapour on the respiratory functions of male Swiss mice exposed to 100 mg/m^3 for two daily periods of 30 min each for 5 weeks. Body weights were not affected. There was a decrease in pulmonary compliance, but no effects were found on pulmonary resistance, respiratory volume, or functional residual capacity. The lungs showed an increase in phospholipid content (Watanabe & Aviado, 1974).

In summary, the toxicological effects on a variety of laboratory animals from repeated inhalation exposure to acrolein vapour at concentrations ranging from 0.39 mg/m^3 to 11.2 mg/m^3 have been studied. Exposure durations ranged from 5 days to as long as 52 weeks. In general, body weight gain reduction, decrement of pulmonary function, and pathological changes in nose, upper airways, and lungs have been documented in most species exposed to acrolein concentrations of 1.6 mg/m^3 or more. Pathological changes include inflammation, metaplasia, and hyperplasia of the respiratory tract. Significant mortality has been observed following repeated exposures to acrolein vapour at concentrations above 9.07 mg/m^3.

7.2.3 Repeated intraperitoneal exposure

Groups of ten intact or adrenalectomized NMRI mice were injected intraperitoneally with saline or acrolein in water at daily doses of 4 to 16 mg/kg body weight for 1 to 6 days. One week after the last injection the mice were killed for autopsy.

Clinical signs of toxicity were hunched posture, inactivity, and ruffled fur. Total body weight and relative thymus and spleen weights showed a dose-related reduction, while the adrenals showed an increase in relative weight. Histologically, thymic necrosis and splenic atrophy were the only changes observed. These changes were absent in controls and in adrenalectomized mice. The levels of reduced glutathione and the activity of glutathione S-transferase in liver cytosol were unchanged, but the rate of glutathione synthesis was increased. Repeated exposure to acrolein caused a progressively less pronounced effect on mortality (Warholm et al., 1984).

7.3 Biochemical effects and mechanisms of toxicity

7.3.1 Protein and non-protein sulfhydryl depletion

A dose-related non-protein sulfhydryl (reduced glutathione) depletion was observed in the nasal respiratory mucosa of male Fischer rats after nose-only exposure for 3 h to acrolein vapour at concentrations of 0.23-11.4 mg/m^3 (McNulty et al., 1984; Lam et al., 1985). Depletion of glutathione in the liver was not observed at these exposure levels (McNulty et al., 1984). The glutathione depletion in the nasal mucosa appeared irreversible at 11.4 mg/m^3 (McNulty et al., 1984). In female C3Hf/HeHa mice, intraperitoneally exposed once to doses between 20 and 80 mg/kg body weight and killed 2 h later, a dose-related decrease in liver glutathione levels was observed. These doses are however extremely high considering the fact that a dose of 4.5 mg/kg body weight was lethal within 1.7 h (Gurtoo et al., 1981a).

A dose-related *in vitro* glutathione depletion has been observed in human bronchial fibroblasts (Krokan et al., 1985), human bronchial epithelial cells (Grafström et al., 1988), human chronic myeloid leukemia cells (Crook et al., 1986b), and human and rat phagocytic cells (Witz et al., 1987) from the lowest acrolein concentration tested (56 µg/litre). The effect has also been reported to occur in isolated rat hepatocytes (Zitting & Heinonen, 1980; Dawson et al., 1984; Dore & Montaldo, 1984; Ku & Billings, 1986) and in rat liver or lung microsomal suspensions (Patel et al., 1984), the lowest-observed-effect level being 1400 µg/litre (Dawson et al., 1984). Ku & Billings (1986) observed that both mitochondrial and cytosolic glutathione levels were decreased.

As a result of acrolein exposure, there was a decrease in the level of both membrane surface and soluble protein sulfhydryl groups in *in vitro* human and rat phagocytic cells (Witz et al., 1987) and a decrease in the level of soluble protein sulfhydryl compounds in human bronchial epithelial cells (Grafström et al., 1988). Acrolein has also been shown to cause a decrease in membrane surface protein sulfhydryl groups in rat hepatocytes (Ku & Billings, 1986) and to reduce the protein sulfhydryl content of liver and lung microsomal preparations (Patel et al., 1984).

7.3.2 Inhibition of macromolecular synthesis

When partially hepatectomized Wistar rats were exposed intraperitoneally to a single acrolein dose of 0.5, 1.6, 2.0, or 2.7 mg/kg body weight, a dose-related inhibition of the synthesis of DNA and RNA was measured in liver and lung cells (Munsch & Frayssinet, 1971).

Inhibition of DNA, RNA, and/or protein synthesis has been observed in *Escherichia coli* (Kimes & Morris, 1971), the slime mold *Physarum polycephalum* (Leuchtenberger et al., 1968), the alga *Dunaliella bioculata* (Marano & Puiseux-Dao, 1982), and in *in vitro* mammalian cells such as mouse kidney cells (Leuchtenberger et al., 1968) and polyoma transformed Chinese hamster cells (Alarcon, 1972). Acrolein was shown to inhibit RNA polymerase in isolated rat liver nuclei (Moule & Frayssinet, 1971) and isolated rat liver DNA polymerase (Munsch et al., 1973). The activity of the latter enzyme is associated with at least one functional sulfhydryl group, and preincubation of the enzyme with 2-mercaptoethanol protected against the inhibitory action of acrolein. Since acrolein did not inhibit isolated *Escherichia coli* polymerase I, devoid of sulfhydryl groups in its active centre, Munsch et al. (1973) suggested that the inhibitory action of acrolein is caused by a reaction with sulfhydryl groups.

7.3.3 Effects on microsomal oxidation

In *in vitro* studies, acrolein has been shown to convert rat liver cytochrome P-450 to cytochrome P-420 and to inhibit rat liver NADPH-cytochrome-*c* reductase (EC 1.6.2.4) in a time- and concentration-related fashion (Marinello et al., 1978; Ivanetich et al., 1978; Berrigan et al., 1980; Gurtoo et al., 1981b; Marinello et al., 1981; Patel et al., 1984; Cooper et al., 1987). A concomitant decrease occurred in the activity of several monooxygenases: benzphetamine *N*-demethylase, aniline hydroxylase, ethylmorphine *N*-demethylase (Patel et al., 1984), and 7-ethoxyresorufin *O*-deethylase (Cooper et al., 1987). The lowest-observed-effect levels reported were 2 mg/litre for inactivation of cytochrome P-450 (Gurtoo et al., 1981b) and 25 mg/litre for inhibition of NADPH-cytochrome-*c* reductase (Marinello et al., 1981). It was also shown that the addition of sulfhydryl-containing agents, such as cysteine, acetylcysteine, glutathione, dithiothreitol, and semicarbazide, reduced the above effects, suggesting that acrolein produces them by reacting with sulfhydryl groups at the active sites.

7.3.4 Other biochemical effects

In vivo studies with Holtzman rats have shown that rat liver alkaline phosphatase (EC 3.1.3.1) and tyrosine aminotransferase (EC 2.6.1.5) activities are increased markedly after inhalation of acrolein for 4 h at a concentration of 14.7 mg/m^3 or after a single intraperitoneal injection of acrolein in water at doses of 1.5-6 mg/kg body weight (Murphy et al., 1964; Murphy, 1965). The increase in alkaline phosphatase activity following intraperitoneal injection was shown to be dose related (Murphy, 1965). The effects were reduced by prior adrenalectomy or hypophysectomy or by pretreatment with protein synthesis inhibitors such as actinomycin D, puromycin, and ethionine, suggesting that the irritant action of acrolein stimulates the pituitary-adrenal system to release glucocorticoids, which act to increase the synthesis of adaptive liver enzymes (Murphy, 1965; Murphy & Porter, 1966). Increased plasma and adrenal levels of corticosterone were measured in Holtzman rats one hour after a single intraperitoneal injection (3 mg/kg body weight) of acrolein in water (Szot & Murphy, 1971). The hypersecretion of glucocorticoids could also explain the observed increase in liver glycogen level following intraperitoneal exposure to acrolein at a dose of 1.5 mg/kg body weight (Murphy & Porter, 1966).

At a concentration of 5.6 mg/litre, acrolein produced an 80% inhibition of the noradrenaline-induced oxygen consumption of isolated hamster brown fat cells (Pettersson et al., 1980). In addition, Zollner (1973) observed an acrolein-induced inhibition of the respiration of intact rat liver mitochondria and found evidence for an inhibition at three different sites: glutamate transport, inorganic phosphorus transport, and the enzyme succinic dehydrogenase (EC 1.3.5.1).

Several sulfhydryl-sensitive enzymes have been shown to be inhibited by acrolein *in vitro*, e.g., rabbit muscle L-lactate dehydrogenase (EC 1.1.1.27), yeast glucose-6-phosphate dehydrogenase (EC 1.1.1.49), and yeast alcohol dehydrogenase (EC 1.1.1.1) (Benedict & Stedman, 1969), porcine lung 15-hydroxyprostaglandin dehydrogenase (EC 1.1.1.141) (Liu & Tai, 1985), rat liver or urothelium S-adenosyl-L-methionine-DNA(cytosine-5)-methyltransferase (EC 2.1.1.37) (Cox et al., 1988), and O^6-methylguanine-DNA methyltransferase (EC 2.1.1.63) in cultured human bronchial fibroblasts (Krokan et al, 1985). In two of these studies glutathione was shown to afford protection against inhibition of the enzyme (Liu & Tai, 1985; Cox et al., 1988).

It has been suggested that the formation of a Schiff base between acrolein and sensitive amine groups is responsible for the observed inhibition *in vitro* of Salmonella typhimurium deoxyribose-5-phosphate aldolase (EC 4.1.2.4) at a concentration of approximately 14 mg/litre (Wilton, 1976) and human plasma α_1-proteinase inhibitor (Gan & Ansari, 1987).

Acrolein was shown to cause a concentration-dependent increase in lipid peroxidation in isolated rat hepatocytes at levels that also decreased glutathione concentrations (Zitting & Heinonen, 1980). Preincubation of washed rat liver microsomes with acrolein abolished the protective effect of glutathione against iron/ascorbate-induced lipid peroxidation (Haenen et al, 1988). The authors claimed that the protective effect of glutathione was mediated by vitamin E scavenging membrane lipid radicals. It was suggested that acrolein was inhibiting a glutathione-dependent reductase enzyme responsible for reducing vitamin E radicals back to vitamin E.

7.4 Immunotoxicity and host resistance

Acrolein has been found to depress pulmonary host defenses in a number of tests.

In female Swiss mice, exposed to measured concentrations of 1.1, 6.9, and 14.2 mg/m^3 for 8 h, a concentration-related increase in the survival of *Staphylococcus aureus* was seen at levels of 6.9 mg/m^3 or more (Astry & Jakab, 1983). A concentration- and time-related increase in the survival of *S. aureus* and *Proteus mirabilis* was found in male Swiss CD-1 mice exposed to measured concentrations of 2.3 to 4.6 mg/m^3 for 24 h. When the mice were also infected with Sendai virus, intrapulmonary bacterial death was further suppressed (Jakab, 1977). An increased survival of *Klebsiella pneumoniae*, but no increased mortality from pneumonia following challenges with *Streptococcus zooepidemicus*, was observed in female CD-1 mice after exposure to acrolein at a measured concentration of 0.23 mg/m^3 for 3 h per day over 5 days (Aranyi et al., 1986). In female CR/CD-1 mice, exposure to a measured acrolein concentration of 4.6 mg/m^3, for one period of 6 h or for 7 consecutive daily periods of 8 h, resulted in an increased mortality from *Streptococcus pyogenes* and Salmonella typhimurium, respectively, but not from influenza A virus (Campbell et al., 1981).

Sherwood et al. (1986) exposed groups of 33 male Sprague-Dawley rats to acrolein vapour at analysed concentrations of 0.39,

2.45 or 6.82 mg/m^3 for 3 weeks (6 h per day and 5 days per week). The relative pulmonary bactericidal activity to *K. pneumoniae* was not affected nor was the number of alveolar cells. However, the number of peritoneal macrophages was decreased at concentrations of 2.45 mg/m^3 or more, and alveolar and peritoneal macrophages had altered phagocytic and enzymic patterns at $\geq$ 0.39 mg/m^3.

When SPF-OFA rats were exposed continuously to a measured acrolein concentration of 1.26 mg/m^3 for 18 days, they exhibited an increased mortality from an infection by *Salmonella enteritidis*. However, no such effect was observed following 63 days of exposure (Bouley et al., 1975).

Acrolein has been shown to inhibit *in vitro* protein synthesis (Leffingwell & Low, 1979), and phagocytosis and ATPase (EC 3.6.1.37-38) activity (Low et al., 1977) in rabbit pulmonary alveolar macrophages. Inhibition of a graft-versus-host reaction in rats was found after Wistar rat spleen cells were incubated *in vitro* with acrolein and injected into all four feet of hybrid F1 rats. In addition, a decreased mitogen response of human peripheral lymphocytes was recorded (Whitehouse et al., 1974). Acrolein was also found to inhibit *in vitro* chemotaxis of human polymorphonuclear leucocytes (Bridges et al., 1977).

7.5 Reproductive toxicity, embryotoxicity, and teratogenicity

Two *in vivo* exposure studies have been reported. In one, 3 male and 21 female SPF-OFA rats were exposed continuously to acrolein vapour at a measured concentration of 1.26 mg/m^3 for 25 days and allowed to mate on day 4. It should be noted that the exposure period did not cover the complete spermatogenic period of 60 days. The number of pregnant animals and the number and mean weight of the fetuses were unaffected in comparison to the control rats (Bouley et al., 1985). In the second study, groups of 12 to 16 New Zealand rabbits were injected (into the ear vein) with a solution of acrolein in saline (3, 4.5 or 6 mg/kg body weight) on the 9th day of gestation. At 4.5 and 6 mg/kg body weight, maternal toxicity was indicated by the death of 3 and 6 dams, respectively, and embryotoxicity by a dose-related increase in resorptions which was significant at 6 mg/kg body weight. It was also reported that the number of malformed and retarded fetuses increased in a dose-related manner, although the increases were statistically non-significant. No effects on maternal toxicity, embryotoxicity or fetuses were noted at 3 mg/kg body weight (Claussen et al., 1980).

A clear effect on the development of the embryo *in vivo* was observed only when acrolein was administered close to the target site by intra-amniotic injection. Using groups of 12 to 19 pregnant New Zealand rabbits, 0, 10, 20, or 40 µl of a 0.84% solution of acrolein in saline was injected into the amnion of all embryos in one of the uterine horns on the 9th day of gestation. The embryos in the other uterine horn received saline only and served as controls. The dams were killed on day 28 of gestation. There was a dose-related increase in the rate of resorptions and malformations, significant at doses of 20 µl or more per embryo. Malformations included deformed and asymmetric vertebrae, spina bifida, deformed and fused ribs, and lack or fusion of sternum segments. No effect was observed on the number of implantations and fetuses or on fetal growth (Claussen et al., 1980). A similar study was carried out on pregnant Sprague-Dawley rats injected with acrolein doses of 0, 0.1, 1.0, 2.5, 5.0, 10.0 or 100 µg per fetus in 10 ml of saline on the 13th day of pregnancy. The dams were killed on day 20 of gestation. A dose-related increase in the percentage of dead and resorbed fetuses per litter was observed at all dose levels. The total number of litters at each dose level varied from 4 to 18. The percentage of malformed fetuses per litter also was increased in a dose-related manner at doses of up to 5 µg per fetus. The increase was significant only up to this dose level, probably because at higher doses there were few surviving fetuses. Treatment-related effects included oedema, micrognathia, hindlimb and forelimb defects, and hydrocephaly (Slott & Hales, 1985). These results confirmed the findings of an earlier, identical test using dose levels of 0.1, 10, and 100 µg per fetus (Hales, 1982).

Acrolein was also shown to be embryotoxic and teratogenic in the rat whole embryo culture system. As with embryos exposed *in vivo*, the concentration range for teratogenicity was very narrow (Slott & Hales, 1986). Schmid et al. (1981) and Mirkes et al. (1984) observed embryotoxicity but no teratogenicity in the same test system, this being probably the result of the different test conditions used (Slott & Hales, 1986). Depletion of glutathione by buthionine sulfoximine enhanced the embryotoxicity and teratogenicity of acrolein in the *in vitro* studies of Slott & Hales (1987a), whereas exogenous glutathione afforded protection against these effects (Slott & Hales, 1987b).

In a mouse limb bud culture system, acrolein induced impairment of limb bud differentiation, indicative of a teratogenic action (Stahlmann et al., 1985). When acrolein was injected into chicken eggs, embryotoxic and teratogenic effects were observed

(Kankaanpaa et al., 1979; Korhonen et al., 1983; Chhibber & Gilani, 1986).

In summary, acrolein can induce teratogenic and embryotoxic effects if administered directly to the embryos or fetuses. However, the fact that no effect was found in rabbits injected intravenously with 3 mg/kg suggests that neither skin contact nor inhalation of acrolein is likely to affect the developing embryo.

7.6 Mutagenicity and related end-points

7.6.1 DNA damage

In vitro studies have revealed interactions between acrolein and DNA and RNA (Munsch et al., 1974b; section 6.2.1). Acrolein has also been found to react with purine and pyrimidine bases or intact DNA *in vitro*, and several adducts have been identified (Descroix, 1972; Hemminki et al., 1980; Lutz et al., 1982; Chung et al., 1984; Shapiro et al., 1986; section 6.2.2.2). Cyclic deoxyguanosine DNA adducts were formed in a dose-dependent fashion in acrolein-exposed Salmonella typhimurium TA100 and TA104. This adduct formation correlated with the induction of reverse mutations in these strains (section 7.6.2; Foiles et al., 1989).

No data on the formation of DNA adducts following exposure of animals to acrolein are available.

Incubation of Fischer-344 rat nasal mucosal homogenate with acrolein resulted in a concentration-dependent increase in DNA-protein cross-linking, which was not observed following inhalation exposure of rats to acrolein at a concentration of 4.6 mg/m^3 for 6 h (Lam et al., 1985). According to the authors this could be explained by the preferential reaction of acrolein with sulfhydryl groups. DNA-protein cross-linking and single strand breaks were observed *in vitro* in human bronchial fibroblasts at cytotoxic concentrations of 1.7 mg/litre or more (Grafström et al., 1986, 1988), and there was indirect evidence for some formation of DNA interstrand cross-linking (Grafström et al., 1988). No DNA-protein or DNA interstrand cross-linking was induced by acrolein in mouse L1210 leukemia cells at cytotoxic levels that produced single strand breaks and/or alkali-labile sites in these cells (Erickson et al., 1980) or in human chronic myeloid leukemia cells (Crook et al., 1986a). In non-mammalian assays, Fleer & Brendel (1982) did not find DNA interstrand cross-linking or single strand breaks in MB1072-2B yeast cells and Kubinski et al. (1981) observed DNA-cell binding in *Escherichia coli* in the presence of a rat liver S9 fraction. These studies demonstrate that effects on DNA occur only at cytotoxic concentrations of acrolein. Results of DNA repair tests are not available. Acrolein has been demonstrated to inhibit O^6-methylguanine-DNA methyltransferase (EC 2.1.1.63.; section 7.3.4) and, therefore, can be expected to reduce the capacity for repair of O^6-guanine alkylations in DNA (Krokan et al., 1985).

7.6.2 Mutation and chromosomal effects

The results of tests for the induction of gene mutations and chromosome damage by acrolein are summarized in Table 10.

In point mutation assays with Salmonella typhimurium, the positive or equivocal responses obtained were all observed within a narrow dose range of up to 10-56 µg per plate, higher doses being toxic. Clearly positive, dose-related increases in revertant colonies per plate at 2-5 times the background rate were observed in the absence of metabolic activation only in TA100 (Lutz et al., 1982; Foiles et al., 1989; Hoffman et al., 1989), TA104 (Marnett et al., 1985; Foiles et al., 1989; Hoffman et al., 1989), and TA98 (Lijinsky & Andrews, 1980). Khudoley et al. (1986) reported positive results in strains TA98 and TA100 without specifying dose levels or revertant rates. Some evidence for indirect mutagenicity was found in strains TA1535 (Hales, 1982) and TA100 (Haworth et al., 1983), the slight increase in TA100 revertants being dose related. However, negative results, both with and without metabolic activation, have also been obtained in these strains. Some of these negative results were clearly related to the incubation conditions, which were probably highly toxic, e.g., those obtained in spot tests (Andersen et al., 1972; Florin et al., 1980). In Salmonella typhimurium TA100 and TA104, strains that show a clear mutagenic response to acrolein, DNA-acrolein adducts have also been identified (section 7.6.1).

Acrolein did not induce sex-linked recessive lethality in *Drosophila melanogaster* adults (Zimmering et al., 1985), but induced a 12-fold increase in sex-linked recessive lethality in hatching eggs and larva at an exposure level that was not reported but caused over 75% larval death (Rapoport, 1948). In the latter test, treatment of adults was reported to be less effective.

Table 10. Tests for gene mutation and chromosomal damage by acrolein

Test description	Organism	Species/strain/cell type	Result[a]	Reference
Gene mutations				
Reverse mutations	bacteria	Salmonella typhimurium TA1535	±(+S9) −	Hales (1982) Florin et al. (1980); Loquet et al. (1981); Haworth et al. (1983); Lijinsky & Andrews (1980)
		Salmonella typhimurium TA100	+(−S9) ±(+S9) −	Lutz et al. (1982); Khudoley et al., 1986; Foiles et al. (1989); Hoffman et al. (1988) Haworth et al. (1983) Florin et al. (1980); Loquet et al. (1981); Basu & Marnett (1984); Lijinsky & Andrews (1980)
		Salmonella typhimurium TA104	+(−S9)	Marnett et al. (1985); Foiles et al. (1989); Hoffman et al. (1989)
		Salmonella typhimurium TA102 Salmonella typhimurium TA98	− +(−S9) −	Marnett et al. (1985) Lijinsky & Andrews (1980); Khudoley et al. (1986) Florin et al. (1980); Loquet et al. (1981); Haworth et al. (1983); Basu & Marnett (1984)
		Salmonella typhimurium TA1537	−	Florin et al. (1980); Haworth et al. (1983); Lijinsky & Andrews (1980)
		Salmonella typhimurium TA1538 Salmonella typhimurium, 8 strains Escherichia coli 343/113 Escherichia coli WP2 uvrA	− − − ±(−S9)	Basu & Marnett (1984); Lijinsky & Andrews (1980) Andersen et al. (1972) Ellenberger & Mohn (1976, 1977)[b] Hemminki et al. (1980)
	yeast yeast	Saccharomyces cerevisiae S211, S138 Saccharomyces cerevisiae N123	− +(−S9)	Izard (1973) Izard (1973)[c]
Forward mutations				

Table 10 (contd).

Test description	Organism	Species/strain/cell type	Result[a]	Reference
Forward mutations	man	normal fibroblasts	-(-S9)	Curren et al. (1988)
	hamster	DNA-repair-deficient fibroblasts	+(-S9)	Curren et al. (1988)
		V79 cells	+(-S9)	Smith et al. (1990)
Sex-linked lethal mutations	insect	*Drosophila melanogaster*, hatching eggs and young larva	+	Rapoport (1948)[d]
		Drosophila melanogaster, adults	-	Zimmering et al. (1985)[e]
Chromosomal damage				
Aberrations	hamster	ovary cells *in vitro*	±(+S9)	Au et al. (1980)
			±(-S9)	Galloway et al. (1987)
Sister chromatid exchanges	hamster	ovary cells *in vitro*	+(-S9)	Au et al. (1980)
			+(-S9)	Galloway et al. (1987)
	man	lymphocytes *in vitro*	+(-S9)	Wilmer et al. (1986)
Dominant lethal mutations (ip exposure)	mouse	germ cells	-	Epstein & Shafner (1968)

[a] + = ≥2 x background rate or statistically significant (P < 0.05); ± = equivocal; - = negative.
[b] Details for this test were not reported.
[c] Plate test for *petite* mutations (production of a respiratory-deficient mutant).
[d] Doses were not reported. Treatment of adults was found to be less effective.
[e] Exposure via feeding solution or via injection.

Three cytogenetic tests have been carried out with acrolein, two in Chinese hamster ovary cells (Au et al., 1980; Galloway et al., 1987) and one in human lymphocytes (Wilmer et al., 1986). Acrolein was shown to induce sister chromatid exchanges in the absence of a metabolic activating system in all three studies. The lowest effective concentration was 56 µg/litre (Galloway et al., 1987). No increase in chromosome aberrations was reported in one study (Galloway et al., 1987), while chromosome breakage was reported in another study at cytotoxic concentrations (Au et al., 1980).

Three properties of acrolein make it difficult to test for mutagenicity: its high cytotoxicity, which prevents the expression of any mutagenic activity, and its high reactivity and volatility, which prevent it reaching the target sites. However, acrolein can be considered to be a weak mutagen in some bacterial and fungal test systems in the absence of metabolic activating systems and to induce sister chromatid exchange in cultured mammalian cells.

7.6.3 Cell transformation

Acrolein (0.4 µg/ml) has been found not to exhibit transforming potential in C3H/10T1/2 cells but to initiate the process of transformation. The latter was measured by exposing cultures to acrolein for 24 h and, subsequently, to a phorbol ester for 6 weeks (Abernethy et al., 1983).

7.7 Carcinogenicity

7.7.1 Inhalation exposure

Inhalation experiments of appropriate duration specifically designed to assess the carcinogenicity of acrolein vapour have not been conducted.

An 81-week study (52 weeks of acrolein exposure at 9.2 mg/m^3 followed by 29 weeks without exposure) on groups of 36 Syrian golden hamsters of both sexes is described in section 7.2.2. The effects of treatment included a persistent and statistically significant reduction in body weight in females, an increased relative brain weight in males and females at 52 weeks, and an increased relative lung weight in females at 52 weeks. Apart from one small tracheal papilloma in an acrolein-exposed female, no respiratory tract tumours were observed in control or treated hamsters (Feron & Kruysse, 1977). In order to elucidate a possible co-carcinogenic action of acrolein, Feron & Kruysse (1977) also exposed groups of 30 Syrian golden hamsters of both sexes to measured acrolein vapour concentrations of 0 or 9.2 mg/m^3, 7 h per day and 5 days per week for 52 weeks, and, for the same period, either weekly to an intratracheal dose of benzo[*a*]pyrene or once every 3 weeks to a subcutaneous dose of diethylnitrosamine. Total dose levels were 18.2 or 36.4 mg benzo[*a*]pyrene and 2.1 µl diethylnitrosamine. Survivors were killed at week 81, and all hamsters were subjected to postmortem examination. The mortality rate in the groups treated with benzo[*a*]pyrene was slightly higher than in other groups. The incidence of benzo[*a*]pyrene-induced respiratory tract tumours was slightly (but statistically insignificantly) higher in females also exposed to acrolein vapour. In these females, at the higher dose level of benzo[*a*]pyrene, respiratory tract tumours occurred earlier and the number of malignant tumours was slightly increased. Taken together, these observations might suggest an enhancing effect of acrolein on benzo[*a*]pyrene carcinogenesis in the respiratory tract, but the effect cannot be considered proven.

In a study by Le Bouffant et al. (1980), rats, 20 animals per group, were exposed to 18.3 mg/m^3, 1 h/day and 5 days/week, for 10 or 18 months. No tumours or metaplasias were found.

7.7.2 Oral exposure

In a study by Lijinsky & Reuber (1987), groups of 20 Fischer-344 rats of both sexes were exposed to weekly prepared acrolein of unspecified purity in drinking-water. Each cage of four rats received 80 ml of acrolein solutions at concentrations of 100 or 250 mg/litre for 124 weeks (males only) or 625 mg/litre for 104 weeks (both sexes) for 5 days per week (this was estimated by the Task Group to be equivalent to approximately 5, 12.5, and 50 mg/kg body weight per day, respectively). Total doses were 1200, 3100, and 6500 mg per rat, respectively. Controls were left untreated. Survivors were killed at week 123-132 and all rats were subjected to postmortem examination. The mean survival time was about 120 weeks for experimental and control groups. There was a marginal, but not statistically significant, increase in the incidence of adrenal cortical adenomas (5/20) in female rats at 625 mg/litre, compared to concurrent controls (1/20), and a decrease in the incidence of pituitary neoplasms in both sexes at 625 mg/litre. In addition, 2 of 20 females given 625 mg/litre had hyperplastic nodules of the adrenal cortex. The authors cited historic control values for adrenal cortical adenomas or carcinomas in female Fischer-344 rats from other laboratories as 1.3% at 26 months of age and 4.8% in a lifespan study. Because of limited numbers of animals used and concerns regarding the purity and stability of acrolein in the dosed drinking-water, the authors of this study did not consider it to be a definitive carcinogenicity bioassay. In addition, the Task Group considered the historical control values quoted by the authors to be of limited use in evaluating the importance of the tumour incidence found in this study.

Acrolein appeared to be too toxic to Syrian golden hamsters following oral exposure by gavage in corn oil to conduct an effective carcinogenicity study (Lijinsky & Reuber, 1987).

7.7.3 Skin exposure

In a study by Salaman & Roe (1956), a group of 15 S strain mice of unspecified sex and age received weekly doses of 0.5% acrolein in acetone for 10 weeks. The total dose was 12.6 mg per rat, although the purity of the acrolein was not reported. The control group comprised 20 mice. From day 25 after the first acrolein treatment, the mice received once per week a skin application of 0.17% croton oil (0.085% in weeks 2 and 3) for 18 weeks. Croton oil and acrolein were applied alternately at 3 or 4 day intervals. At the end of treatment, the mortality rate and the incidence of skin papillomata were similar to those of the controls treated only with croton oil. However, this study must be considered inadequate because of the limited number of animals used and the short duration of the experiment.

7.8 Interacting agents

Free sulfhydryl-containing compounds have been found to give protection against the adverse effects of acrolein *in vitro*, e.g., the inhibition of enzymes involved in macromolecular synthesis (Munsch et al., 1973), liver microsomal cytochrome P-450s (Marinello et al., 1978; Berrigan et al., 1980; Gurtoo et al., 1981b, Patel et al., 1984; Cooper et al., 1987), and several other sulfhydryl-sensitive enzymes (Liu & Tai, 1985; Cox et al., 1988), the adverse effects on rabbit alveolar macrophages (Low et al., 1977; Leffingwell & Low, 1979), and the impairment of mouse limb bud differentiation (Stahlmann et al., 1985). Free sulfhydryl-containing agents protected against the acute lethal effects of acrolein in Charles River rats (Sprince et al., 1979) and in DBA/2J mice (Gurtoo et al., 1981a).

When Swiss-Webster mice were exposed to acrolein-formaldehyde mixtures, the percentage decrease in respiratory rate was found to be less than the sum of the percentage decreases due to each compound alone (Kane & Alarie, 1978). In acrolein-exposed Fischer-344 rats, pretreatment with formaldehyde resulted in a lower percentage decrease in respiratory rate compared to non-pretreated rats (Babiuk et al., 1985). It was suggested in both investigations that acrolein and formaldehyde competed for the same receptor (competitive agonism). In a comparable experiment, the maximum percentage decrease in the respiratory rate of Swiss-Webster mice exposed to a mixture of acrolein and sulfur dioxide was lower than that of acrolein alone. This antagonistic effect was thought to be caused by a chemical reaction in the air phase between the two compounds, which reduced the effective concentrations (Kane & Alarie, 1979).

In Fischer-344 rats exposed to formaldehyde vapour (7.4 mg/m^3) once for 6 h, co-exposure to acrolein vapour (4.6 mg/m^3) resulted in a higher increase in DNA-protein cross-linking than was observed with formaldehyde alone. Acrolein alone did not increase DNA-protein cross-linking in this experiment (Lam et al., 1985).

In a study by Hales et al. (1988), anaesthetized, artificially ventilated mongrel dogs were exposed to acrolein or hydrochloric acid with added synthetic smoke composed of carbon particles for 10 min. The dogs were exposed to smoke with or without analytically determined acrolein concentrations of < 458 mg/m^3, 458-687 mg/m^3 or > 687 mg/m^3. Smoke with acrolein, but not smoke with hydrochloric acid, produced non-cardiogenic, peribronchiolar pulmonary oedema in a concentration- and time-related fashion. Both acrolein and hydrochloric acid produced airway damage consisting of mucosal degeneration and desquamation and inflammatory cell infiltration. Acrolein at levels above 458 mg/m^3 also caused fibrin deposition in the alveolar spaces that juxtaposed injured bronchioles.

8. EFFECTS ON HUMANS

8.1 Single exposure

8.1.1 Poisoning incidents

One man was exposed dermally and by inhalation when acrolein was sprayed into his face following an accident in a chemical plant. Immediately, his face and eyelids were burnt. Within 20 h he was hospitalized with fever, cough, frothy sputum, cyanosis, and acute respiratory failure. Two months after the accident, the opening of the right bronchus was obstructed and the upper trachea showed slight oedema with haemorrhagic spots. At 18 months he had developed chronic bronchitis and emphysema, which might have been a sequel of the accidental exposure (Champeix et al., 1966).

One case of attempted oral suicidal intoxication has been reported. The man swallowed approximately 1.5 g of acrolein in a glass of orange juice. Blood was found in his stomach and the number of red and white blood cells was increased. Gastroscopic examination showed shrinkage of the stomach and a massive chronic gastritis with erosions and ulceration. Further examination of the stomach revealed regenerating mucous membranes, few mucous glands, granulation and scarring of the serosa, shrinkage and stenosis of the pylorus, lymphadenitis, and haemosiderin deposition in lymph nodes. The man was successfully treated by gastrectomy (Schielke, 1987).

Two cases of suspected exposure to acrolein have been reported. The death of two young boys who inhaled smoke from an overheated frier for approximately 2 h was thought to be related to acrolein exposure, although other chemicals might also have been involved. One of the boys was found dead, while the other suffered from acute respiratory failure. Following oxygen therapy, the second boy died due to asphyxia. At autopsy a massive cellular desquamation of the bronchial lining was observed. The tracheal and bronchial lumina were filled with debris and the lungs showed multiple infarcts (Gosselin et al., 1979).

Four female factory workers operating a machine for cutting and sealing polyethylene bags and a fifth sitting next to the machine complained of a burning sensation in the eyes, a feeling of dryness and irritation in the nose and throat, and itching and irritation of the skin of the face, neck and forearms. These complaints were related to the smoke developed. The presence of formaldehyde and "acrolein and/or other aldehydes" in the smoke was suspected and confirmed. During heavy smoke exposure, itching eruptions developed on exposed skin. Drowsiness and headache was also experienced. All symptoms were reversible (Hovding, 1969).

8.1.2 Controlled experiments

8.1.2.1 Vapour exposure

Several studies with volunteers have been conducted with the object of establing thresholds for odour perception and recognition and for effects on the eyes, nose, respiratory tract, and nervous system. The results of these studies are summarized in Table 11. The exposure period was up to 60 min. In most cases the concentration of acrolein was determined colorimetrically, although a few reports did not include a description of the analytical method (Plotnikova, 1957; Sinkuvene, 1970; Harada, 1977). Sinkuvene (1970) reported the threshold for changes in the electrical activity of the brain cortex, as measured by electro-encephalography, to be 0.05 mg/m^3. However, this result cannot be evaluated since experimental data were not provided. The odour perception threshold for sensitive people was 0.07 mg/m^3.

In studies by Weber-Tschopp et al. (1977), groups of human volunteer students of both sexes were exposed either for 60 min to acrolein at a concentration of 0.69 mg/m^3 or to gradually increasing acrolein concentrations from 0 up to 1.37 mg/m^3 over 35 min followed by a 5-min exposure to 1.37 mg/m^3. In further experiments with side-stream cigarette smoke instead of pure acrolein vapour, it was noted that the effects of pure acrolein vapour were small compared to those produced by side-stream smoke with the same acrolein vapour concentration. It was concluded that acrolein was only to a minor extent responsible for the effects observed (Weber-Tschopp et al., 1976). It must be noted, however, that a significant part of the acrolein in side-stream cigarette smoke may be associated with particulate matter (Ayer & Yeager, 1982) and would not have been measured. This may have resulted in an underestimation of the acrolein concentration in the smoke. Many of the studies considered in this section are old and the analytical techniques are often poorly described; the absolute figures reported may, therefore, be suspect.

Table 11. Thresholds for acute effects of acrolein on humans

Concentration (mg/m³)	Exposure period (min)	Effect	Reference
0.05		changes in electrical activity of brain cortex	Sinkuvene (1970)
0.07		odour perception by most sensitive individuals	Sinkuvene (1970)
0.13	5	no or medium subjective eye irritation	Darley et al. (1960)[a]
0.21	5	increased incidence of subjective eye irritation	Weber-Tschopp et al. (1977)[b]
0.34	10	increased incidence of subjective nasal irritation	Weber-Tschopp et al. (1977)[b]
0.34	30	time-related increase in eye-blink frequency	van Eick (1977)[a]
0.39	10	increased incidence of subjective annoyance	Weber-Tschopp et al. (1977)[b]
0.48		odour recognition	Leonardos et al. (1969)
0.59	15	increase in eye-blink frequency	Weber-Tschopp et al. (1977)[b]
0.6	10	increase in sensitivity to light	Plotnikova (1957)
0.69	40	decrease in respiratory rate; increased incidence of subjective general irritation of eyes, nose, and neck	Weber-Tschopp et al. (1977)[c]
0.69	10	increase in eye-blink frequency	Weber-Tschopp et al. (1977)[c]
1	3	slight subjective conjunctival irritation	Plotnikova (1957)
1	3	stinging sensation in nose	Plotnikova (1957)
1.1	5	increased incidence of subjective eye irritation	Stephens et al. (1961)[a]
1.1	5	increase in tear volume, pH, and lysozyme activity	Harada (1977)
1.37	35	decrease in respiratory rate	Weber-Tschopp et al. (1977)[b]
1.5	3	pneumographic changes in rhythm and amplitude of respiratory movements	Plotnikova (1957)

Table 11 (contd).

Concentration (mg/m³)	Exposure period (min)	Effect	Reference
1.7	3	reflex action on optical chronaxy	Plotnikova (1957)
1.88		extreme subjective irritation of all exposed mucosae; lacrimation within 20 seconds	Sim & Pattle (1957)
2.80		extreme subjective irritation of all exposed mucosae; lacrimation within 5 seconds	Sim & Pattle (1957)
3	5	medium to severe subjective eye irritation	Darley et al. (1960)[a]
4	2-3	acute subjective conjunctival and nasal irritation; painful sensation in nasopharyngeal region	Plotnikova (1957)

[a] exposure of eyes only
[b] exposure to gradually increasing concentrations up to 1.37 mg/m³
[c] exposure to a fixed concentration

8.1.2.2 Dermal exposure

In an investigation into irritant dermatitis possibly caused by contaminants present in diallylglycol carbonate monomer, patch tests were conducted with acrolein in ethanol at concentrations of 0.01, 0.1, 1, and 10% on groups of 8, 10, 48, and 20 volunteers, respectively. At 1%, six positive reactions were recorded, four cases of serious oedema with bullae and two of erythema. At 10%, all subjects showed positive reactions with bullae, necrosis, inflammatory cell infiltrate, and papillary oedema (Lacroix et al., 1976).

8.2 Long-term exposure

No data are available on the long-term exposure of humans to acrolein.

9. EFFECTS ON OTHER ORGANISMS IN THE LABORATORY AND FIELD

9.1 Aquatic organisms

A summary of acute aquatic toxicity data is presented in Table 12. In most of these studies, the amount of acrolein added was reported but the concentrations present were not measured. In these cases, the actual concentrations may have been lower than the nominal ones in view of the volatility of the substance and its hydration rate (see section 4.2).

One of the studies in Table 12 (Lorz et al., 1979) is a comparatively detailed examination of the acute toxicity of acrolein to Coho salmon. Within 144 h of exposure to 0.075 mg/litre or more, all fish died. In surviving fish the activity of gill Na^+,K^+-ATPase (EC 3.6.1.37) and the tolerance to subsequent sea-water exposure were not affected at concentrations up to 0.05 mg/litre. A histological examination of the gills, kidneys, and liver at 0, 0.05, and 0.1 mg/litre revealed concentration-dependent adverse effects.

A 3-generation 64-day test with the crustacean *Daphnia magna* was conducted in a flow-through open system with well water at 20 °C, a pH between 7.0 and 7.3, a dissolved oxygen concentration of 7.5 mg/litre, and a water hardness of 35 mg $CaCO_3$/litre. The highest concentration that did not result in mortality was 0.0169 mg/litre (acrolein concentrations were measured in this study). Survival was reduced at levels of 0.0336 mg/litre or more, but the number of young per female was not affected even at the highest concentration tested, 0.0427 mg/litre (Macek et al., 1976).

Macek et al. (1976) also reported on a 60-day test with fathead minnow (*Pimephales promelas*) in a flow-through open system with well water at 25 °C, a pH between 6.6 and 6.8, a dissolved oxygen concentration of 8.2 mg/litre, and a water hardness of 32 mg $CaCO_3$/litre. The highest concentration without adverse effects was 0.0114 mg/litre (acrolein concentrations were measured in this study). At 0.0417 mg/litre, there was increased mortality among offspring. No adverse effects were found on survival and mortality of adults, number of spawnings and number of eggs per female, number of eggs per spawn, length of offspring, or hatchability.

Table 12. Acute aquatic toxicity of acrolein

Organism	Species	Temperature (°C)	pH	Dissolved O_2 (mg/litre)	Hardness (mg $CaCO_3$ per litre)	Stat/flow open/closed[a]	Exposure period	Parameter[b]	Concentration (mg/litre)	Reference
Fresh water										
alga	*Enteromorpha intestinalis*	25				stat, closed	24 h	50% inhibition of photosynthesis	1.8[c]	Fritz-Sheridan (1982)
alga	*Cladophora glomerata*	25				stat, closed	24 h	50% inhibition of photosynthesis	1.00[c]	Brown & Fowler (1967)
alga	*Anabaena*	25				stat, closed	24 h	50% inhibition of photosynthesis	0.69[c]	Bringmann & Kuhn (1977)
bacterium	*Proteus vulgaris*	37	7.0			stat, closed	2 h	50% growth reduction	0.02	Bringmann (1978)
bacterium	*Pseudomonas putida*	25	7.0			stat, closed	16 h	TT	0.21	Bringmann et al. (1980)
protozoan	*Entosiphon sulcatum*	25	6.9			stat, closed	72 h	TT	0.85	Bringmann & Kuhn (1980)
protozoan	*Chilomonas paramecium*	20	6.9			stat, closed	48 h	TT	1.7	Bringmann & Kuhn (1980)
protozoan	*Uronema parduczi*	25	6.8			stat, closed	20 h	TT	0.44	Unrau et al. (1965)[d]
mollusc	snail (*Bulinus truncatus*)	21-25				flow, open	48 h	99-100% mortality	20-25	Ferguson et al. (1961)
mollusc	snail (*Biomphalaria glabrata*), eggs					stat, open	3 h / 24 h	100% mortality / 10% mortality	10 / 1.25	Ferguson et al. (1961)
mollusc	snail (*Biomphalaria glabrata*), adults					stat, open	24 h / 24 h	98% mortality / 35% mortality	10 / 2.5	Ferguson et al. (1961)

Table 12 (contd).

Organism	Species	Temperature (°C)	pH	Dissolved O_2 (mg/litre)	Hardness (mg $CaCO_3$ per litre)	Stat/flow open/closed[a]	Exposure period	Parameter[b]	Concentration (mg/litre)	Reference
crustacean	water flea (*Daphnia magna*)	20	7.0–7.3	7.5	35	stat, open	48 h	LC_{50}	0.057	Macek et al. (1976)
crustacean	water flea (*Daphnia magna*)	22	7.0–8.2		154	stat, closed	48 h	EC_{50}[f]	0.093	Randall & Knopp (1980)
crustacean	water flea (*Daphnia magna*)	22	7.4–9.4	6–9	173	stat, closed	48 h	LC_{50}	0.083	LeBlanc (1980)
fish	harlequin fish (*Rasbora heteromorpha*)	20	7.2		20	flow, open	48 h	LC_{50}	0.06	Alabaster (1969)
fish	fathead minnow (*Pimephales promelas*)	25	6.6–6.8	8.2	32	flow, open	144 h	LC_{50}	0.084	Macek et al. (1976)[e]
fish	golden orfe (*Leuciscus idus melanotus*)	20	7–8	≥ 5	200–300	stat	48 h	LC_{50}	0.25 & 2.5	Juhnke & Ludemann (1978)
fish	goldfish (*Carassius auratus*)	20	6–8	≥ 4	108	stat, open	24 h	LC_{50}	< 0.08	Bridie et al. (1979)[c,e]
fish	Bluegill sunfish (*Leopomis macrochirus*)	21–23	6.5–7.9	10–0.3	32–48	stat, closed	96 h	LC_{50}	0.09	Buccafusco et al. (1981)
fish	Coho salmon (*Oncorhynchus kisutch*)	10	7.4–7.6	> 10	100	stat, open	96 h	LC_{50}	0.068	Lorz et al. (1979)[g]

Table 12 (contd).

Organism	Species	Temperature (°C)	pH	Dissolved O_2 (mg/litre)	Hardness (mg $CaCO_3$ per litre)	Stat/flow open/closed[a]	Exposure period	Parameter[b]	Concentration (mg/litre)	Reference
Marine										
mollusc	common mussel (*Mytilus edulis*)	15				stat, closed	6 h 6 h 8 h	40% mortality 70% mortality 70% detached mussels	0.6 1.0 0.57	Rijstenbil & van Galen (1981)[e,h]

[a] static or flow-through test, open or closed system
[b] TT = toxic threshold for inhibition of cell multiplication
[c] exposure to Magnacide-H (92% acrolein, 8% inert ingredients)
[d] field study, resurgence of snails was delayed by 8 to 12 months
[e] analysis for acrolein was reported
[f] the effect was complete immobilization
[g] static-renewal test
[h] static-renewal test (1.6% salinity)

It is clear from Table 12 why acrolein is also used as an algicide, slimicide, and molluscicide.

9.2 Terrestrial organisms

9.2.1 Birds

The LD_{50} for the adult starling (*Sturnus vulgaris*) was reported to be > 100 mg/kg body weight. The birds were observed for 7 days after dosing, but only two birds per dose were tested (Schafer, 1972).

9.2.2 Plants

Acrolein is used as biocide, particularly to control aquatic plants such as *Elodea canadensis*, *Vallisneria spiralis* (ribbonweed), and *Potamogeton tricarinatus* (floating pondweed). In Australia, a maximum concentration of about 15 mg/litre over a period not exceeding a few hours has been imposed. In the USA, acrolein is injected into larger channels over longer periods at low concentrations (approximately 0.1 mg/litre over 48 h) (Bowmer & Sainty, 1977). It has been shown that the dosage of acrolein required for control, as defined by the product of time and concentration required for 80% reduction in biomass, is independent of the separate values of concentration and time, provided that the concentration exceeds 0.1 mg/litre and the dosage exceeds 2 mg/litre per h. In tank experiments, the minimum dosages required for 80% control of ribbonweed and floating pondweed were about 4 and 26 mg/litre per h, respectively (Bowmer & Sainty, 1977). The effective dosage (> 80% kill) for *Elodea canadensis* was 8 to 10 mg/litre per h (Van Overbeek et al., 1959; Bowmer & Smith, 1984). Sublethal concentrations of acrolein stimulated the growth of *Elodea* (Bowmer & Smith, 1984).

Elongation of pollen tubes of lily seeds (*Lilium longiflorum*) was inhibited completely after a 5-h exposure to acrolein vapour at a measured concentration of 0.91 mg/m^3, a temperature of 28 °C, and a relative humidity of 60%. A 10% inhibition was found after 1 h (Masaru er al., 1976).

The nature and extent of adverse effects on various crops grown in soil irrigated by acrolein-treated water have been investigated in two studies. Acrolein concentrations varied between 15 and 50 mg/litre of supply water. Most furrow-irrigated crops, including beans, clover, corn, and millet, did not show any damage. Significant damage to foliage was observed in cotton at acrolein concentrations of 25 mg/litre or more, but there was no evidence of chronic or residual phytotoxicity. Slight damage to the foliage of cucumbers and tomatoes was observed at 40 mg/litre. Vegetable seedlings in contact with treated water were damaged even at the lowest concentrations used (Unrau et al., 1965; Ferguson et al., 1965).

10. EVALUATION OF HUMAN HEALTH RISKS AND EFFECTS ON THE ENVIRONMENT

10.1 Evaluation of human health risks

10.1.1 Exposure

Exposure of the general population to acrolein occurs mainly via air. Exposure via water would only be significant in cases of ingestion of, or skin contact with, acrolein deliberately applied as a biocide to irrigation water. Oral exposure to acrolein may also occur via alcoholic beverages or heated foodstuffs (chapters 3 and 5).

In urban areas, average levels of up to 15 $\mu g/m^3$ and maximum levels of up to 32 $\mu g/m^3$ have been measured away from industrial sources. Near industries and close to the exhaust pipes of vehicles, engines, and combustion appliances, levels ten to one hundred times higher may occur. Extremely high levels of acrolein in the mg/m^3 range can be found as a result of fires (section 5.2.1).

Major indoor sources of acrolein are combustion appliances and tobacco smoking (section 3.2.4). Levels of acrolein in smoke from indoor open fires for cooking or heating purposes have not been reported. Smoking one cigarette per m^3 of room-space in 10-13 min has been shown to lead to acrolein vapour concentrations of 450-840 $\mu g/m^3$ (section 5.2.1). Recent occupational exposure levels of acrolein in the air at sites of its production or processing are not available. Workplace levels of over 1000 $\mu g/m^3$ have been reported in situations involving the heating of organic materials (section 5.3).

In summary, the main source of exposure of the general population to acrolein is via tobacco smoke. General environmental pollution by vehicle exhaust and the smoke of burning organic materials is the next most important source.

10.1.2 Health effects

Owing to the reactivity of acrolein, retention at the site of entry into the body, usually the respiratory tract, is high (section 6.1). Primary pathological findings are limited principally to these sites (sections 7 and 8). Any acrolein absorbed is liable to react directly with protein and non-protein sulfhydryl groups or with primary and secondary amines such as those found in proteins and nucleic acids (sections 6.2 and 7.3). Acrolein may also be metabolized to mercapturic acids, acrylic acid, glycidaldehyde or glyceraldehyde (section 6.3). Evidence for the last three metabolites has only been obtained *in vitro*.

Acrolein is a cytotoxic agent (section 7.1.5) highly toxic to experimental animals and man following acute exposure via different routes (sections 7.1.1 and 8.1.1). The vapour is very irritating to the eyes and the respiratory tract. Liquid acrolein is a corrosive substance. The no-observed-adverse-effect level for irritant dermatitis from ethanolic acrolein was found to be 0.1% (section 8.1.2.2). The odour perception threshold for the most sensitive individuals is reported to be 0.07 mg/m^3 (8.1.2.1). Experiments with human volunteers show a lowest-observed-adverse-effect level of 0.13 mg/m^3, at which level eyes may become irritated after 5 min. In addition to irritation of the eyes, changes in respiratory tract function are evident at or above 0.7 mg/m^3 (40-min exposure) (section 8.1.2.1). At higher concentrations, degeneration of the respiratory epithelium and irritation of all exposed mucosa develop. Oedematous changes in the tracheal and bronchial mucosa and bronchial obstruction can be expected after very high exposure to acrolein vapour (section 8.1).

There are no human toxicological data from long-term exposure to acrolein. The toxicity from exposure to acrolein vapour has been relatively well investigated in several animal studies for exposure periods of up to 52 weeks (section 7.2). Both respiratory tract function and histopathological effects have been observed at 0.5-0.8 mg/m^3 (continuous exposure). Toxicological effects in the respiratory tract have been documented in most animal species exposed repeatedly to acrolein concentrations of 1.6-3.2 mg/m^3 or more, and mortality has occurred following exposure to concentrations above 9 mg/m^3. There is limited evidence that acrolein can depress pulmonary host defenses in mice and rats.

Acrolein can induce teratogenic and embryotoxic effects if administered directly into the amnion. However, the fact that no effect was found in rabbits injected intravenously with 3 mg/kg suggests that human exposure to acrolein is unlikely to affect the developing embryo (section 7.5).

Acrolein has been shown to interact with DNA and RNA *in vitro* and to inhibit their synthesis both *in vivo* and *in vitro*. *In vitro*, it induces gene mutations in bacteria and fungi and sister chromatid exchanges in mammalian cells (section 7.6). There is inadequate evidence to allow the mutagenic potential in humans to be assessed reliably.

One long-term drinking-water study with rats (130 weeks) and two inhalation tests, one with hamsters (81 weeks) and the other with rats (40 or 70 weeks), failed to demonstrate carcinogenic or clear co-carcinogenic effects of acrolein (section 7.7). Due to the shortcomings of the tests used, acrolein cannot be considered to have been adequately tested for carcinogenicity and no conclusions concerning its carcinogenicity are possible.

The threshold levels of acrolein that cause irritation and health effects are 0.07 mg/m^3 for odour perception, 0.13 mg/m^3 for eye irritation, 0.3 mg/m^3 for nasal irritation and eye blinking, and 0.7 mg/m^3 for decreased respiratory rate. Since the level of acrolein rarely exceeds 0.030-0.040 μg/m^3 in polluted urban air or smoke-filled restaurants, acrolein alone is unlikely to reach annoyance or harmful levels in normal circumstances. Provided that acrolein concentrations are maintained below 0.05 mg/m^3, most of the population will be spared from any known annoyance or health effects. However, in polluted urban areas and smoke-filled rooms, acrolein is present in combination with other irritating aldehydes, and control of acrolein alone is not sufficient to prevent annoyance or harmful effects.

10.2 Evaluation of effects on the environment

Acrolein is released into the environment during production of the compound itself and its derivatives, in processes involving incomplete combustion and/or pyrolysis of organic substances, by photochemical oxidation of specific air pollutants, and through biocidal use, spills, and waste disposal (chapter 3).

Degradation in the atmosphere begins mainly by reaction with hydroxyl radicals. The calculated atmospheric residence time is approximately one day (section 4.2). Photolysis does not occur to a significant degree (section 4.2.1). In natural water, acrolein dissipates fairly rapidly as a result of catalysed hydration, reactions with organic material, and volatilization (sections 4.2 and 4.3). Acrolein has a low soil adsorption potential (section 4.1). Aerobic and anaerobic biodegradation of the compound has been reported, although its toxicity to microorganisms may prevent biodegradation (section 4.3.1). Based on its physical and chemical properties, bioaccumulation would not be expected to occur (section 4.3.2). It can be concluded that acrolein is unlikely to persist in any environmental compartment.

Acrolein is very toxic to aquatic organisms. Acute EC_{50} or LC_{50} values for various species range between 0.02 and 2.5 mg/litre. The 60-day NOAEL for fish (fathead minnow) is 0.0114 mg/litre (section 9.1).

In view of the high toxicity of acrolein to aquatic organisms, the substance presents a risk to aquatic life at or near sites of industrial discharges, spills, and biocidal use.

11. FURTHER RESEARCH

a) Human exposure characteristics should be further evaluated. This applies to exposure due to environmental and occupational air, as well as to intake from food and beverages.

b) These evaluations should include determinations of other chemicals that occur with acrolein and that interact or have biological effects similar to those due to acrolein exposure.

c) The most important target organ for airborne acrolein exposure is the respiratory system. Therefore, further studies including epidemiological studies should focus on this system and particularly on the occupational environment. Possible decreases in host resistance to respiratory infections should be investigated.

d) The uptake of acrolein in the different parts of the respiratory system should be examined further. The metabolism and excretion of acrolein, as well as of its metabolites from the respiratory system, should be given high priority as there is an almost total lack of information about these processes.

e) The efficacy of sulfhydryl compounds, such as N-acetylcysteine or 2-mercaptoethylsulfonic acid sodium salt (MESNA) as antidotes for acrolein poisoning should be evaluated.

12. PREVIOUS EVALUATIONS BY INTERNATIONAL BODIES

Evidence for the potential carcinogenicity of acrolein has been evaluated by the International Agency for Research on Cancer (IARC, 1979, 1985, 1987). The evidence for carcinogenicity was considered to be inadequate both in animals and in humans. Thus no evaluation could be made of the carcinogenicity of acrolein to humans.

Regulatory standards established by national bodies in various countries and the EEC are summarized in the data profile of the International Register of Potentially Toxic Chemicals (IRPTC, 1990) and are tabulated in the Health and Safety Guide for Acrolein (WHO, 1991).

REFERENCES

ABERNETHY, D.J., FRAZELLE, J.H., & BOREIKO, C.J. (1983) Relative cytotoxicity and transforming potential of respiratory irritants in the C3H/10T1/2 cell transformation system. Environ. Mutagen., 5: 419 (abstract).

ALABASTER, J.S. (1969) Survival of fish in 164 herbicides, insecticides, fungicides, wetting agents, and miscellaneous substances. Int. Pest Control, 11: 29-35.

ALARCON, R.A. (1968) Fluorometric determination of acrolein and related compounds with m-aminophenol. Anal. Chem., 40: 1704-1708.

ALARCON, R.A. (1972) Acrolein, a component of a universal cell-growth regulatory system: a theory. J theor. Biol., 37: 159-167.

ALARCON, R.A. (1976) Formation of acrolein from various amino-acids and polyamines under degradation at 100 °C. Environ. Res., 12: 317-326.

ALTSHULLER, A.P. & BUFALINI, J.J. (1965) Photochemical aspects of air pollution: a review. Photochem. Photobiol., 4: 97-146.

ALTSHULLER, A.P. & MCPHERSON, S.P. (1963) Spectrophotometric analysis of aldehydes in the Los Angeles atmosphere. J. Air Pollut. Control Assoc., 13: 109-111.

ANDERSEN, K.J., LEIGHTY, E.G., & TAKAHASHI, M.T. (1972) Evaluation of herbicides for possible mutagenic properties. J. agric. food Chem., 20: 649-656.

ANDERSSON, K., HALLGREN, C., LEVIN, J.-O., & NILSSON, C.-A. (1981) Solid chemosorbent for sampling sub-ppm levels of acrolein and glutaraldehyde in air. Chemosphere, 10: 275-280.

ARANYI, C., O'SHEA, W.J., GRAHAM, J.A., & MILLER, F.J. (1986) The effects of inhalation of organic chemical air contaminants on murine lung host defenses. Fundam. appl. Toxicol., 6: 713-720.

ARTHO, A. & KOCH, R. (1969) [The concentration of acrolein and hydrogen cyanide in cigarette smoke]. Mitt. Lebensm. Hyg. (Bern), 60: 379-388 (in German).

ASTRY, C. & JAKAB, G.J. (1983) The effects of acrolein exposure on pulmonary antibacterial defenses. Toxicol. appl. Pharmacol., 67: 49-54.

ATKINSON, R., ASCHMANN, S.M., WINER, A.M., & PITTS, J.N. (1981) Rate constants for the gas-phase reactions of O_3 with a series of carbonyls at 296 K. Int. J. chem. Kinet., 13: 1133-1150.

ATKINSON, R., ASCHMANN, S.M., & PITTS, J.N. (1983) Kinetics of the gas-phase reactions of OH radicals with a series of α,β-unsaturated carbonyls at 299 + 2 K. Int. J. chem. Kinet., 15: 75-81.

ATKINSON, R., ASCHMANN, S.M., & GOODMAN, M.A. (1987) Kinetics of the gas-phase reactions of NO_3 radicals with a series of alkynes, haloalkenes, and α,β-unsaturated aldehydes. Int. J. chem. Kinet., 19: 299-307.

References

AU, W., SOKOVA, O.I., KOPNIN, B., & ARRIGHI, F.E. (1980) Cytogenetic toxicity of cyclophosphamide and its metabolites *in vitro*. Cytogenet. cell Genet., **26**: 108-116.

AYER, H.E. & YEAGER, D.W. (1982) Irritants in cigarette smoke plumes. Am. J. public Health, **72**: 1283-1285.

BABIUK, C., STEINHAGEN, W.H., & BARROW, C.S. (1985) Sensory irritation response to inhaled aldehydes after formaldehyde pretreatment. Toxicol. appl. Pharmacol., **79**: 143-149.

BAKER, R.R., DYMOND, H.F., & SHILLABEER, P.K. (1984) Determination of α,β-unsaturated compounds formed by a burning cigarette. Anal. Proc. (Lond.), **21**: 135-137.

BALLANTYNE, B., DODD, D.E., PRITTS, I.M., NACHREIMER, D.J., & FOWLER, E.H. (1989) Acute vapour inhalation toxicity of acrolein and its influence as a trace contaminent in 2-methoxy-3,4-dihydro-2H-pyran. Hum. Toxicol., **8**: 229-235.

BARROWS, M.E., PETROCELLI, S.R., MACEK, K.J., & CARROLL, J.J. (1980) Bioconcentration and elimination of selected water pollutants by bluegill sunfish (*Lepomis macrochirus*). In: Proceedings of the 1978 Symposium on dynamics, exposure and hazard assessment of toxic chemicals, Ann Arbor, Michigan, Ann Arbor Science, pp. 379-392.

BARTLEY, T.R. & GANGSTAD, E.O. (1974) Environmental aspects of aquatic plant control. J. Irrig. Drain. Div., **100**: 231-244.

BASU, A.K. & MARNETT, L.J. (1984) Molecular requirements for the mutagenicity of malondialdehyde and related acroleins. Cancer Res., **44**: 2848-2854.

BEAUCHAMP, R.O., ANDJELKOVICH, D.A., KLIGERMAN, A.D., MORGAN, K.T., & HECK, H. d'A. (1985) A critical review of the literature on acrolein toxicity. CRC crit. Rev. Toxicol., **14**: 309-380.

BEELEY, J.M., CROW, J., JONES, J.G., MINTY, B., LYNCH, R.D., & PRYCE, D.P. (1986) Mortality and lung histopathology after inhalation lung injury. The effect of corticosteroids. Am. Rev. respir. Dis., **133**: 191-196.

BEN-DYKE, R., SANDERSON, D.M., & NOAKES, D.N. (1970) Acute toxicity data for pesticides. World Rev. Pest. Control, **9**: 119-127.

BENEDICT, R.C. & STEDMAN, R.L. (1969) Composition studies on tobacco. XXXVII. Inhibition of lactic, alcohol and glucose-6-phosphate dehydrogenases by cigarette smoke and components thereof. Tob. Sci., **13**: 166-168.

BERRIGAN, M.J., GURTOO, H.L., SHARMA, S.D., STRUCK, R.F., & MARINELLO, A.J. (1980) Protection by N-acetylcysteine of cyclophosphamide metabolism - related *in vivo* depression of mixed function oxygenase activity and *in vitro* denaturation of cytochrome P-450. Biochem. biophys. Res. Commun., **93**: 797-803.

BIGNOZZI, C.A., CHIORBOLI, C., MALDOTTI, A., & CARASSITI, V. (1980). Atmospheric reactivity of 1,3-butadiene - nitrogen monoxide and acrolein - nitrogen monoxide systems. Ann. Chim. (Rome), **70**: 453-461.

BOETTNER, E.A. & BALL, G.L. (1980). Thermal degradation products from PVC film in food-wrapping operations. Am. Ind. Hyg. Assoc. J., **41**: 513-522.

BOHMANN, J.-J. (1985) [Aging behaviour of beer.] Monatsschr. Brauwiss., 4: 175-180 (in German).

BOOR, P.J. & ANSARI, G.A.S. (1986) High-performance liquid chromatographic method for quantitation of acrolein in biological samples. J. Chromatogr., 375: 159-164.

BOULEY, G., DUBREUIL, A., GODIN, J., & BOUDENE, C. (1975) Effets, chez le rat, d'une faible dose d'acroléine inhalée en continu. Eur. J. Toxicol., 8: 291-297.

BOWMER, K.H. & HIGGINS, M.L. (1976) Some aspects of the persistence and fate of acrolein herbicide in water. Arch.environ. Contam. Toxicol., 5: 87-96.

BOWMER, K.H. & SAINTY, G.R. (1977) Management of aquatic plants with acrolein. J. aquat. Plant Manage., 15: 40-46.

BOWMER, K.H. & SMITH, G.H. (1984) Herbicides for injection into flowing water: acrolein and endothal-amine. Weed Res., 24: 201-211.

BOWMER, K.H., LANG, A.R.G., HIGGINS, M.L., PILLAY, A.R., & TCHAN, Y.T. (1974) Loss of acrolein from water by volatilization and degradation. Weed Res., 14: 325-328.

BOYLAND, E. & CHASSEAUD, L.F. (1967) Enzyme-catalysed conjugations of glutathione with unsaturated compounds. Biochem. J., 104: 95-102.

BRIDGES, R.B., KRAAL, J.H., HUANG, L.J.T., & CHANCELLOR, M.B. (1977) Effects of cigarette smoke components on *in vitro* chemotaxis of human polymorphonuclear leukocytes. Infect. Immun., 16: 240-248.

BRIDIE, A.L., WOLFF, C.J.M., & WINTER, M. (1979a) BOD and COD of some petrochemicals. Water Res., 13: 627-630.

BRIDIE, A.L., WOLFF, C.J.M., & WINTER, M. (1979b) The acute toxicity of some petrochemicals to goldfish. Water Res., 13: 623-626.

BRINGMANN, G. (1978) [Determination of the harmful biological action of water-endangering substances on protozoa; I. Bacteria fed flagellates.] Z. Wasser-Abwasser Forsch., 11: 210-215 (in German).

BRINGMANN, G. & KUHN, R. (1977) [Limiting values of the harmful action of water-endangering substances on bacteria (*Pseudomonas putida*) and green algae (*Scenedesmus quadricauda*) in the cell multiplication inhibition test.] Z. Wasser-Abwasser Forsch., 10: 87-98 (in German).

BRINGMANN, G. & KUHN, R. (1980) [Determination of the harmful biological action of water-endangering substances on protozoa; II. Bacteria fed ciliates.] Z. Wasser-Abwasser Forsch., 13: 26-31 (in German).

BRINGMANN, G., KUHN, R., & WINTER, A. (1980) [Determination of the harmful biological action of water-endangering substances on protozoa; III Saprozoic flagellates.] Z. Wasser-Abwasser Forsch., 13: 170-173 (in German).

BROWN, P.W. & FOWLER, C.A. (1967) The toxicity of tobacco smoke solutions to *Proteus vulgaris*. Beitr. Tabakforsch., 4: 78-83.

BUCCAFUSCO, R.J., ELLS, S.J., & LEBLANC, G.A. (1981) Acute toxicity of priority pollutants to Bluegill (*Lepomis macrochirus*). Bull. environ. Contam. Toxicol., 26: 446-452.

BUCKLEY, L.A., JIANG, X.Z., JAMES, R.A., MORGAN, K.T., & BARROW, C.S. (1984) Respiratory tract lesions induced by sensory irritants at the RD_{50} concentration. Toxicol. appl. Pharmacol., 74: 417-429.

CAMPBELL, D.N. & MOORE, R.H. (1979) The quantitative determination of acrylonitrile, acrolein, acetonitrile and acetone in workplace air. Am. Ind. Hyg. Assoc. J., 40: 904-909.

CAMPBELL, K.I., GEORGE, E.L., & WASHINGTON, I.S. (1981) Enhanced susceptibility to infection in mice after exposure to dilute exhaust from light duty diesel engines. Environ. Int., 5: 377-382.

CANTONI, C., BIANCHI, M.A., RENON, P., & CALCINARDI, C. (1969) [Bacterial and chemical alterations during souring in salted pork.] Atti. Soc. Ital. Sci. Vet., 23: 752-756 (in Italian).

CARPENTER, C.P., SMYTH, H.F., POZZANI, U.C. (1949) The assay of acute vapor toxicity, and the grading and interpretation of results on 96 compounds. J. ind. Hyg. Toxicol., 31: 343-346.

CATILINA, P., THIEBLOT, L., & CHAMPEIX, J. (1966) Lesions respiratoires expérimentales par inhalation d'acroléine chez le rat. Arch. Mal. prof. Méd. Trav. Sécur. soc. (Paris), 27: 857-867.

CHAMPEIX, J., COURTIAL, L., PERCHE, E., & CATILINA, P. (1966) Broncho-pneumopathie aiguë par vapeurs d'acroléine. Arch. Mal. prof. Méd. Trav. Sécur. Soc., 27: 794-796.

CHAVIAMO, A.H., GILL, W.B., RUGGIERO, U.J., & VERMEULEN, C.W. (1985) Experimental cytoran cystitis and prevention by acetylcysteine. J. Urol., 134: 598-600.

CHHIBBER, G. & GILANI, S.H. (1986) Acrolein and embryogenesis: an experimental study. Environ. Res., 39: 44-49.

CHOU, W.L., SPEECE, R.E., & SIDDIQI, R.H. (1978) Acclimation and degradation of petrochemical wastewater components by methane fermentation. Biotechnol. Bioeng. Symp., 8: 391-414.

CHRAIBER, L.B., SOSNOVSKY, S.I., TATARKIN, Y.N., & VINNIKOVA, L.I. (1964) [Air pollution with acrolein vapors in expeller and forepress shops of butter and fat mills of Uzbekistan.] Gig. Tr. prof. Zabol., 1(11): 49-50 (in Russian).

CHUNG, F.-L., YOUNG, R., & HECHT, S.S. (1984) Formation of cyclic $1,N^2$-propanodeoxyguanosine adducts in DNA upon reaction with acrolein or crotonaldehyde. Cancer Res., 44: 990-995.

CLAUSSEN, U., HELLMANN, W., & PACHE, G. (1980) The embryotoxicity of the cyclophosphamide metabolite acrolein in rabbits, tested *in vivo* by i.v. injection and by the yolk-sac method. Drug Res., 30: 2080-2083.

COHEN, I.R. & ALTSHULLER, A.P. (1961) A new spectrophotometric method for the determination of acrolein in combustion gases and in the atmosphere. Anal. Chem., 33: 726-733.

COOMBER, J.W. & PITTS, J.N. (1969) Molecular structure and photochemical reactivity. XII. The vapor-phase photochemistry of acrolein at 3130 A. J. Am. Chem. Soc., 91: 547-550.

COOPER, K.O., WITMER, C.M., & WITZ, G. (1987) Inhibition of microsomal cytochrome c reductase activity by a series of α,β-unsaturated aldehydes. Biochem. Pharmacol., 36: 627-631.

COSTA, D.L., KUTZMAN, R.S., LEHMANN, J.R., & DREW, R.T. (1986) Altered lung function and structure in the rat after subchronic exposure to acrolein. Am. Rev. respir. Dis., 133: 286-291.

COX, R., GOORHA, S., & IRVING, C.C. (1988) Inhibition of DNA methylase activity by acrolein. Carcinogenesis, 9: 463-465.

CRANE, C.R., SANDERS, D.C., ENDECOTT, B.R., & ABBOTT, J.K. (1986) Inhalation toxicology: VII. Times to incapacitiation and death for rats exposed continuously to atmospheric acrolein vapor, Washington, D.C., Federal Aviation Administration, Office of Aviation Medicine (DOT/FAA/AM-86/5)

CROOK, T.R., SOUHAMI, R.L., & MCLEAN, A.E.M. (1986a) Cytotoxicity, DNA cross-linking, and single strand breaks induced by activated cyclophosphamide and acrolein in human leukemia cells. Cancer Res., 46: 5029-5034.

CROOK, T.R., SOUHAMI, R.L., WHYMAN, G.D., & MCLEAN, A.E.M. (1986b) Glutathione depletion as a determinant of sensitivity of human leukemia cells to cyclophosphamide. Cancer Res., 46: 5035-5038.

CURREN, R.D., YANG, L.L., CONKLIN, P.M., GRAFSTROM, R.C., & HARRIS, C.C. (1988) Mutagenesis of xeroderma pigmentosum fibroblasts by acrolein. Mutat. Res., 209: 17-22.

DAHLGREN, S.E., DALEN, H., & DALHAMM, T. (1972) Ultrastructural observations on chemically induced inflammation in guinea pig trachea. Virchows Arch. Abt. B Zellpathol., 11: 211-223.

DALHAMN, T. & ROSENGREN, A. (1971) Effect of different aldehydes on tracheal mucosa. Arch. Otolarygnol., 83: 496-500.

DARLEY, E.F., MIDDLETON, J.T., & GARBER, M.J. (1960) Plant damage and eye irritation from ozone-hydrocarbon reactions. J. agric. food Chem., 8: 483-485.

DAVIS, T.R.A., BATTISTA, S.P., & KENSLER, C.J. (1967) Mechanism of respiratory effects during exposure of guinea pigs to irritants. Arch. environ. Health, 15: 412-419.

DAWSON, J.R., NORBECK, K., ANUNDI, I., & MOLDEUS, P. (1984) The effectiveness of N-acetylcysteine in isolated hepatocytes, against the toxicity of paracetamol, acrolein, and paraquat. Arch. Toxicol., 55: 11-15.

DEBETHIZY, J.D., UDINSKY, J.R., SCRIBNER, H.E., & FREDERICK, C.B. (1987) The disposition and metabolism of acrylic acid and ethyl acrylate in male Sprague-Dawley rats. Fundam. appl. Pharmacol., **8**: 549-561.

DESCROIX, H. (1972) Etude complémentaire des interactions entre acroléine et cytidine-monophosphate. C. R. Acad. Sci. Paris, **D274**: 2362-2365.

DGEP (1988) Unpublished Review of literature data on acrolein, Leidschendam, The Netherlands, Ministry of Housing, Physical Planning and Environment, Directorate-General of Environmental Protection.

DIAZ MAROT, A., GASSIOT MATAS, M., & FERRER MARTIN, M. (1983) [Stripping and high performance liquid chromatography in the analysis of carbonyl compounds in beers at ppb level.] Afinidad, **40**: 21-24 (in Spanish).

DORE, M. & MONTALDO, C. (1984) [Study on the conjungation *in vitro* of allyl alcohol and its metabolites with reduced glutathione.] Boll. Soc. Ital. Biol. Sper., **60**: 1497-1501 (in Italian).

DRAMINSKI, W., EDER, E., & HENSCHLER, D. (1983) A new pathway of acrolein metabolism in rats. Arch. Toxicol., **52**: 243-247.

EASLEY, D.M., KLEOPFER, R.D., & CARASEA, A.M. (1981) Gas chromatographic-mass spectrometric determination of volatile organic compounds in fish. J. Assoc. Off. Anal. Chem., **64**: 653-656.

EDNEY, E.O., MITCHELL, S., & BUFALINI, J.J. (1982) Atmospheric chemistry of several toxic compounds, Research Triangle Park, North Carolina, US Environmental Protection Agency, Atmospheric Chemistry and Physics Division, Environmental Sciences Research Laboratory, Office of Research and Development (EPA-600/3-82-092, PB 83-146340).

EDNEY, E.O., KLEINDIENST, T.E., & CORSE, E.W. (1986a) Room temperature rate constants for the reaction of OH with selected chlorinated and oxygenated hydrocarbons. Int. J. chem. Kinet., **18**: 1355-1371.

EDNEY, E.O., SHEPSON, P.B., KLEINDIENST, T.E. & CORSE, E.W. (1986b) The photooxidation of allyl chloride. Int. J. chem. Kinet., **18**: 597-608.

EGLE, J.L. (1972) Retention of inhaled formaldehyde, propionaldehyde, and acrolein in the dog. Arch. environ. Health, **25**: 119-124.

EGLE, J.L. & HUDGINS, P.M. (1974) Dose-dependent sympathomimetic and cardioinhibitory effects of acrolein and formaldehyde in the anesthetized rat. Toxicol. appl. Pharmacol., **28**: 358-366.

ELLENBERGER, J. & MOHN, G.R. (1976) Comparative mutagenicity testing of cyclphosphamide and some of its metabolites. Mutat. Res., **37**: 120 (abstract).

ELLENBERGER, J. & MOHN, G.R. (1977) Mutagenic activity of major mammalian metabolites of cyclophosphamide toward several genes of *Escherichia coli*. J. Toxicol. environ. Health, **3**: 637-650.

EPSTEIN, S.S. & SHAFNER H. (1968) Chemical mutagens in the human environment. Nature (Lond.), **219**: 385-387.

ERICKSON, L.C., RAMONAS, L.M., ZAHARKO, D.S., & KOHN, K.W. (1980) Cytotoxicity and DNA cross-linking activity of 4-sulfidocyclophosphamides in mouse leukemia cells *in vitro*. Cancer Res., **40**: 4216-4220.

ESTERBAUER, H., ZOLLNER, H., & SCHOLZ, N. (1975) Reaction of glutathione with conjugated carbonyls. Z. Naturforsch., **30**: 466-473.

FACCHINI, M.C., CHIAVARI, G., & FUZZI, S. (1986) An improved HPLC method for carbonyl compound speciation in the atmospheric liquid phase. Chemosphere, **15**: 667-674.

FERGUSON, F.F., RICHARDS, C.S., & PALMER, J.R. (1961) Control of *Australorbis glabratus* by acrolein in Puerto Rico. Public Health Rep., **76**: 461-468.

FERGUSON, F.F., DAWOOD, I.K., & BLONDEAU, R. (1965) Preliminary field trials of acrolein in the Sudan. Bull. World Health Organ., **32**: 243-248.

FERON, V.J. & KRUYSSE, A. (1977) Effects of exposure to acrolein vapor in hamsters simultaneously treated with benzo[a]pyrene or diethylnitrosamine. J. Toxicol. environ. Health, **3**: 379-394.

FERON, V.J., KRUYSSE, A., TIL, H.P., & IMMEL, H.R. (1978) Repeated exposure to acrolein vapour: subacute studies in hamsters, rats and rabbits. Toxicology, **9**: 47-57.

FISCHER, T., WEBER, A., & GRANDJEAN, E. (1978) [Air pollution due to tobacco smoke in restaurants.] Int. Arch. occup. environ. Health, **41**: 267-280 (in German).

FLEER, R. & BRENDEL, M. (1982) Toxicity, interstrand cross-links and DNA fragmentation induced by 'activated' cyclophosphamide in yeast: comparative studies on 4-hydroperoxy-cyclophosphamide, its monofunctional analogue, acrolein, phosphoramide mustard, and non-nitrogen mustard. Chem.-biol. Interact., **39**: 1-15.

FLORIN, I., RUTBERG, L., CURVALL, M., & ENZELL, C.R. (1980) Screening of tobacco smoke constituents for mutagenicity using the Ames' test. Toxicology, **18**; 219-232.

FOILES, P.G., AKERKAR, S.A., & CHUNG, F.-L. (1989) Application of an immunoassay for cyclic acrolein deoxyguanosine adducts to assess their formation in DNA of *Salmonella typhimurium* under conditions of mutation induction by acrolein. Carcinogenesis, **10**: 87-90.

FRACCHIA, M.F., SCHUETTE, F.J., & MUELLER, P.K. (1967) A method for sampling and determination of organic carbonyl compounds in automobile exhaust. Environ. Sci. Technol., **1**: 915-922.

FRITZ-SHERIDAN, R.P. (1982) Impact of the herbicide Magnacide-H (2-propenal) on algae. Bull. environ. Contam. Toxicol., **28**: 245-249.

GALLOWAY, S.M., ARMSTRONG, M.J., REUBEN, C., COLMAN, S., BROWN, B., CANNON, C., BLOOM, A.D., NAKAMURA, F., AHMED, M., DUK, S., RIMPO, J., MARGOLIN, B.H., RESNICK, M.A., ANDERSON, B., & ZEIGER, E. (1987)

Chromosome aberrations and sister chromatid exchanges in Chinese hamster ovary cells: evaluations of 108 chemicals. Environ. mol. Mutagen., 10(supplement): 1-175.

GAN, J.C. & ANSARI, G.A.S. (1987) Plausible mechanism of inactivation of plasma α_1-proteinase inhibitor by acrolein. Res. Commun. chem. Pathol. Pharmacol., 55: 419-422.

GIUSTI, D.M., CONWAY, R.A., & LAWSON, C.T. (1974) Activated carbon adsorption of petrochemicals. J. Water Pollut. Control Fed., 46: 947-965.

GOSSELIN, B., WATTEL, F., CHOPIN, C., DEGAND, P., FRUCHART, J.C., VAN DER LOO, D., & CRASQUIN, O. (1979) Intoxication aiguë par l'acroléine, une observation. Nouv. Presse méd., 8: 2469-2472.

GRAEDEL, T.E., FARROW, L.A., & WEBER, T.A. (1976) Kinetic studies of the photochemistry of the urban atmosphere. Atmos. Environ., 10: 1095-1116.

GRAFSTROM, R.C., CURREN, R.D., YANG, L.L., & HARRIS, C.C. (1986) Aldehyde-induced inhibition of DNA repair and potentiation of N-nitrosocompound-induced mutagenesis in cultured human cells. Prog. clin. biol. Res., 209A: 255-264.

GRAFSTROM, R.C., DYPBUKT, J.M., WILLEY, J.C., SUNDQVIST, K., EDMAN, C., ATZORI, L., & HARRIS, C.C. (1988) Pathobiological effects of acrolein in cultured human bronchial epithelial cells. Cancer Res., 48: 1717-1721.

GREENHOFF, K. & WHEELER, R.E. (1981) Analysis of beer carbonyls at the part per billion level by combined liquid chromatography and high pressure liquid chromatography. J. Inst. Brew., 86: 35-41.

GREY, T.C. & SHRIMPTON, D.H. (1966) Volatile components of raw chicken breast muscle. Br. poult. Sci., 8: 23-33.

GROSJEAN, D. & WRIGHT ,B. (1983) Carbonyls in urban fog, ice fog, cloudwater and rainwater. Atmos. Environ., 17: 2093-2096.

GUERIN, M.R., OLERICH, G., & HORTON, A.D. (1974) Routine gas chromatographic component profiling of cigarette smoke for the identification of biologically significant constituents. J. chromatogr. Sci., 12: 385-391.

GUICHERIT, R. & SCHULTING, F.L. (1985) The occurrence of organic chemicals in the atmosphere of The Netherlands. Sci. total Environ., 43: 193-219.

GUILLERM, R., BADRE, R., & HEE, J. (1967a) Détermination du seuil d'action des polluants irritants de l'atmosphère - Comparaison de deux méthodes. Ann. occup. Hyg., 10: 127-133.

GUILLERM, R., SAINDELLE, A., FALTOT, P., & HEE, J. (1967b) Action de la fumée de cigarette et de quelques-uns de ses constituants sur les resistances ventilatoires chez le cobaye. Arch. int. Pharmacodyn. Ther., 167: 101-114.

GURTOO, H.L., HIPKENS, J.H., & SHARMA, S.D. (1981a) Role of glutathione in the metabolism-dependent toxicity and chemotherapy of cyclophosphamide. Cancer Res., 41: 3584-3591.

GURTOO, H.L., MARINELLO, A.J., STRUCK, R.F., PAUL, B., & DAHMS, R.P. (1981b) Studies on the mechanism of denaturation of cytochrome P-450 by cyclophosphamide and its metabolites. J. biol. Chem., 256: 11691-11701.

GUSEV, M.I., SVECHNIKOVA, A.I., DRONOV, I.S., GREBENSKOVA, M.D., & GOLOVINA, A.I. (1966) [Substantiation of the daily average maximum permissible concentration of acrolein in the atmosphere.] Gig. i Sanit., 31: 9-13 (in Russian).

HAENEN, G.R.M.M., VERMEULEN, N.P.E., TAI TIN TSOI, J.N.L., RAGETLI, H.M.N., TIMMERMAN, H., & BAST, A. (1988) Activation of the microsomal glutathione-S-transferase dependent protection against lipid peroxidation by acrolein. Biochem. Pharmacol., 37: 1933-1938.

HALES, B.F. (1982) Comparison of the mutagenicity and teratogenicity of cyclophosphamide and its active metabolites, 4-hydroxycyclophosphamide, phosphoramide mustard, and acrolein. Cancer Res., 42: 3016-3021.

HALES, C.A., BARKIN, P.W., JUNG, W., TRAUTMAN, E., LAMBORGHINI, D., HERRIG, N., & BURKE, J. (1988) Synthetic smoke with acrolein but not HCL produces pulmonary edema. J. appl. Physiol., 64: 1121-1133.

HALL, R.H., & STERN, E.S. (1950) Acid-catalysed hydration of acraldehyde. Kinetics of the reaction and isolation of β-hydroxypropaldehyde. J. Chem. Soc., 1950: 490-498.

HARADA, M. (1977) [Biochemical analysis of tear fluid in photochemical smog.] Nippon Ganka Gakkai Zasshi, 81: 275-286 (in Japanese).

HARKE, H.-P., BAARS, A., FRAHM, B., PETERS, H., & SCHULTZ, C. (1972) [On the problem of passive smoking. Relation between the concentration of smoke constituents in the air of several large rooms and the number of smoked cigarettes and time.] Int. Arch. Arbeitsmed., 29: 323-339 (in German).

HAWLEY, G.G. (1981) The condensed chemical dictionary, 10th ed., New York, Van Nostrand Reinhold Co.

HAWORTH, S., LAWLOR, T., MORTELMANS, K., SPECK, W., & ZEIGER, E. (1983) Salmonella mutagenicity test results for 250 chemicals. Environ. Mutagen., Suppl. 1: 3-142.

HAYASE, F., CHUNG, T.-Y., & KATO, H. (1984) Changes of volatile components of tomato fruits during ripening. Food Chem., 14: 113-124.

HEMMINKI, K., FALCK, K., & VAINIO, H. (1980) Comparison of alkylation rates and mutagenicity of directly acting industrial and laboratory chemicals. Arch. Toxicol., 46: 277-285.

HESS, L.G., KURTZ, A.N., & STANTON, D.B. (1978) Acrolein and derivatives. In: Kirk, R.E. & Othmer, D.F. ed. Encyclopedia of chemical technology, 3rd ed., New York, Wiley Interscience, Vol 1: pp. 277-297.

HODGE, H.C. & STERNER, J.H. (1943) Tabulation of toxicity classes. Ind. Hyg. Q., 10: 93-96.

HOFFMAN, C., BASTIAN, H., WIEDENMANN, M., DEININGER, C., & EDER, E. (1989) Detection of acrolein congener-DNA adducts isolated from cellular systems. Arch. Toxicol., Suppl. **13**: 219-223.

HOFFMANN, D., BRUNNEMANN, K.D., GORI, G.B., & WYNDER, E.L. (1975) On the carcinogenicity of marijuana smoke. Recent Adv. Phytochem., **9**: 63-81.

HOLMBERG, B. & MALMFORS, T. (1974) The cytotoxicity of some organic solvents. Environ. Res., **7**: 183-192.

HOSHIKA, Y. & TAKATA, Y. (1976) Gas chromatographic separation of carbonyl compounds as their 2,4-dinitrophenylhydrazones using glass capillary columns. J. Chromatogr., **120**: 379-389.

HOVDING, G. (1969) Occupational dermatitis from pyrolysis products of polythene. Acta dermatovenereol, **49**: 147-149.

HRDLICKA, J. & KUCA, J. (1965) The changes of carbonyl compounds in the heat-processing of meat. Poult. Sci., **44**: 7-31.

HUGOD, C., HAWKINS, L.H., & ASTRUP, P. (1978) Exposure of passive smokers to tobacco smoke constituents. Int. Arch. occup. environ. Health, **42**: 21-29.

IARC (1979) Some monomers, plastics and synthetic elastomers, and acrolein, Lyons, International Agency for Research on Cancer, pp. 479-495 (IARC Monographs on the Evaluation of the Carcinogenic Risk of Chemicals to Man, Vol. 19).

IARC (1985) Allyl compounds, aldehydes, epoxides and peroxides, Lyons, International Agency for Research on Cancer, pp. 133-161 (IARC Monographs on the Evaluation of the Carcinogenic Risk of Chemicals to Man, Vol. 36).

IRPTC (1985) Treatment and disposal methods for waste chemicals, Geneva, International Register of Potentially Toxic Chemicals, United Nations Environment Programme.

IRPTC (1990) Data profile on acrolein, Geneva, International Register of Potentially Toxic Chemicals, United Nations Environment Programme.

IVANETICH, K.M., LUCAS, S., MARSH, J.A., ZIMAN, M.R., KATZ, I.D., & BRADSHAW, J.J. (1978) Organic compounds - Their interaction with and degradation of hepatic microsomal drug-metabolizing enzymes *in vitro*. Drug Metab. Disp., **6**: 218-225.

IZARD, C. (1973) Effets de l'acroléine sur la division cellulaire, le cycle et la synthèse de l'ADN, chez *Vicia faba*. C. R. Acad. Sci. Paris Ser. D, **276**: 1745-1747.

IZARD, C. & LIBERMANN, C. (1978) Acrolein. Mutat. Res., **47**: 115-138.

IZMEROV, N.F., ed. (1984) Acrolein. Moscow, Centre of International Projects, GKNT, 15 pp (IRPTC Scientific Reviews of Soviet Literature on Toxicity and Hazards of Chemicals 50).

JACOBS, W.A. & KISSINGER, P.T. (1982) Determination of carbonyl 2,4-dinitrophenylhydrazones by liquid chromatography/electrochemistry. J. liq. Chromatogr., **5**: 669-676.

JAKAB, G.J. (1977) Adverse effect of a cigarette smoke component, acrolein, on pulmonary defenses and on viral-bacterial interactions in the lung. Am. Rev. respir. Dis., 115: 33-38.

JERMINI, C., WEBER, A., & GRANDJEAN, E. (1976) [Quantitative determination of several gas-phase components of side-stream smoke of cigarettes in indoor air as contribution towards the problem of passive smoking.] Int. Arch. occup. environ. Health, 36: 169-181 (in German).

JONSSON, A. & BERG, S. (1983) Determination of low-molecular-weight oxygenated hydrocarbons in ambient air by cryogradient sampling and two-dimensional gas chromatography. J. Chromatogr., 279: 307-322.

JOUSSERANDOT, P., GREMAIN, J., & DU BOISTESSELIN, R. (1981) L'utilisation de méthodes histologiques pour la démonstration de l'activite anti-inflammatoire de la fusafungine. Sem. Hop. Paris, 57: 143-150.

JUHNKE, I. & LUDEMANN, D. (1978) [Results of examination of 200 chemical compounds for acute toxicity towards fish by means of the goldfish test.] Z. Wasser-Abwasser Forsch., 11: 161-164 (in German).

KANE, L.E. & ALARIE, Y. (1977) Sensory irritation to formaldehyde and acrolein during single and repeated exposures in mice. Am. Ind. Hyg. Assoc. J., 38: 509-521.

KANE, L.E. & ALARIE, Y. (1978) Evaluation of sensory irritation from acrolein-formaldehyde mixtures. Am Ind. Hyg. Assoc. J., 39: 270-274.

KANE, L.E. & ALARIE, Y. (1979) Interactions of sulfur dioxide and acrolein as sensory irritants. Toxicol. appl. Pharmacol., 48: 305-315.

KANKAANPAA, J., ELOVAARA, E., HEMMINKI, K., & VAINIO, H. (1979) Embryotoxicity of acrolein, acrylonitrile and acrylamide in developing chick embryos. Toxicol. Lett., 4: 93-96.

KANTEMIROVA, A.E. (1975) [The disease incidence rate, including temporal disability of workers engaged in the production of acrolein and methylmercaptopropione (MMP) aldehyde.] Trans. Volgograd med. Inst., 26(4): 79-85 (in Russian).

KANTEMIROVA, A.E. (1977) [The disease incidence rate, involving temporal disability of workers engaged in the production of acrolein and MMP aldehyde.] Trans. Volgograd med. Inst., 27(5): 32-33 (in Russian).

KATZ, M. (1977) Methods of air sampling and analysis, 2nd ed., Washington, DC, American Public Health Association.

KAYE, C.M. (1973) Biosynthesis of mercapturic acids from allyl alcohol, allyl esters and acrolein. Biochem. J., 134: 1093-1101.

KERR, J.A. & SHEPPARD (1981) Kinetics of the reactions of hydroxyl radicals with aldehydes studied under atmospheric conditions. Environ. Sci. Technol., 15: 960-963.

KHUDOLEY, V.V., MIZGIREV, I.V., & PLISS, G.B. (1986) [Evaluation of mutagenic activity of carcinogens and other chemical agents with *Salmonella typhimurium* assays.] Vopr. Onkol., 32: 73-80 (in Russian).

KILBURN, K.H. & MCKENZIE, W.N. (1978) Leukocyte recruitment to airways by aldehyde-carbon combinations that mimic cigarette smoke. Lab. Invest., **38**: 134-142.

KIMES, B.W. & MORRIS, D.R. (1971) Inhibition of nucleic acid and protein synthesis in *Escherichia coli* by oxidized polyamines and acrolein. Biochim. Biophys. Acta, **228**: 235-244.

KISSEL, C.L., BRADY, J.L., GUERRA, A.M., PAU, J.K., ROCKIE, B.A., & CASERIO, F.F. (1978) Analysis of acrolein in aged aqueous media. Comparison of various analytical methods with bioassays. J. agric. food Chem., **26**: 1338-1343.

KLOCHKOVSKII, S.P., LUKASHENKO, R.D., PODVYSOTSKII, K.S., & KAGRAMANYAN, N.P. (1981) [Acrolein and formaldehyde content in the air of quarries.] Bezoppasnost. Tr. Prom-St. **1981**(12):38 (in Russian).

KOERKER, R.L., BERLIN, A.J., & SCHNEIDER, F.H. (1976) The cytotoxicity of short-chain alcohols and aldehydes in cultured neuroblastoma cells. Toxicol. appl. Pharmacol., **37**: 281-288.

KORHONEN, A., HEMMINKI, K., & VAINIO, H. (1983) Embryotoxic effects of acrolein, methylacrylates, guanidines and resorcinol on three day chicken embryos. Acta pharmacol. toxicol., **52**: 95-99.

KRILL, R.M. & SONZOGNI, W.C. (1986) Chemical monitoring of Wisconsin's groundwater. J. Am. Water Works Assoc., **78**: 70-75

KROKAN, H., GRAFSTROM, R.C., SUNDQVIST, K., ESTERBAUER, H., & HARRIS, C.C. (1985) Cytotoxicity, thiol depletion and inhibition of O^6-methylguanine-DNA methyltransferase by various aldehydes in cultured human bronchial fibroblasts. Carcinogenesis, **6**: 1755-1759.

KROST, K.J., PELLIZZARI, E.D., WALBURN, S.G., & HUBBARD, S.A. (1982) Collection and analysis of hazardous organic emissions. Anal. Chem., **54**: 810-817.

KRUYSSE, A. (1971) Acute inhalation toxicity of acrolein in hamsters, Zeist, The Netherlands, Central Institute for Nutrition and Food Research, TNO (Report No. R3516).

KU, R.H. & BILLINGS, R.E. (1986) The role of mitochondrial glutathione and cellular protein sulfhydryls in formaldehyde toxicity in glutathione-depleted rat hepatocytes. Arch. Biochem. Biophys., **247**: 183-189.

KUBINSKI, H., GUTZKE, G.E., & KUBINSKI, Z.O. (1981) DNA-cell-binding (DCB) assay for suspected carcinogens and mutagens. Mutat. Res., **89**: 95-136.

KUTZMAN, R.S., MEYER, G.-J., & WOLF, A.P. (1982) The biodistribution and metabolic fate of [^{11}C]-acrylic acid in the rat after acute inhalation exposure or stomach intubation. J. Toxicol. environ. Health, **10**: 969-979.

KUTZMAN, R.S., WEHNER, R.W., & HABER, S.B. (1984) Selected responses of hypertension sensitive and resistant rats to inhaled acrolein. Toxicology, **31**: 53-65.

KUTZMAN, R.S., POPENOE, E.A., SCHMAELER, M., & DREW, R.T. (1985) Changes in rat lung structure and composition as a result of subchronic exposure to acrolein. Toxicology, **34**: 139-151.

KUWATA, K., UEBORI, M., YAMASAKI, H., KUGE, Y., & KISO, Y. (1983) Determination of aliphatic aldehydes in air by liquid chromatography. Anal. Chem., **55**: 2013-2016.

LACROIX, M., BURCKEL, H., FOUSSEREAU, J., GROSSHANS, E., CAVELIER, C., LIMASSET, J.C., DUCOS, P., GRADINSKI, D., & DUPRAT, P. (1976) Irritant dermatitis from diallylglycol carbonate monomer in the optical industry. Contact dermatitis, **2**: 183-195.

LAM, C.-W., CASANOVA, M., & HECK, H.D'A. (1985) Depletion of nasal mucosal glutathione by acrolein and enhancement of formaldehyde-induced DNA-protein cross-linking by simultaneous exposure to acrolein. Arch. Toxicol., **58**: 67-71.

LEACH, P.W., LENG, L.J., BELLAR, T.A., SIGSBY, J.E., & ALTSHULLER, A.P. (1964) Effects of HC/NO_x ratios on irradiated auto exhaust, part II. J. Air Pollut. Control Assoc., **14**: 176-183.

LEACH, C.L., HATOUM, N.S., RATAJCZAK, H.V., & GERHART, J.M. (1987) The pathologic and immunologic effects of inhaled acrolein in rats. Toxicol. Lett., **39**: 189-198.

LEBLANC, G.A. (1980) Acute toxicity of priority pollutants to water flea (*Daphnia magna*). Bull. environ. Contam. Toxicol., **24**: 684-691.

LE BOUFFANT, L., MARTIN, J.C., DANIEL, H., HENIN, J.P., & NORMAND, C. (1980) Action of intensive cigarette smoke inhalations on the rat lung. Role of particulate and gaseous cofactors. J. Natl Cancer Inst., **64**: 273-281.

LEFFINGWELL, C.M. & LOW, R.B. (1979) Cigarette smoke components and alveolar macrophage protein synthesis. Arch. environ. Health, **34**: 97-102.

LENCREROT, P., PARFAIT, A., & JOURET, C. (1984) Rôle des corynebactéries dans la production d'acroléine (2-propenal) dans les rhums. Ind. aliment. agric., **101**: 763-765.

LEONARDOS, G., KENDALL, D., & BARNARD, N. (1969) Odor threshold determinations of 53 odorant chemicals. J. Air Pollut. Control Assoc., **19**: 91-95.

LEUCHTENBERGER, C., SCHUMACHER, M., & HADIMANN, T. (1968) Further cytological and cytochemical studies on the biological significance of the gas phase of fresh cigarette smoke. Z. Präventivmed., **13**: 130-141.

LEVAGGI, D.A. & FELDSTEIN, M. (1970) The determination of formaldehyde, acrolein, and low molecular weight aldehydes in industrial emissions on a single collection sample. J. Air Pollut. Control Assoc., **20**: 312-313.

LIES, K.-H., POSTULKA, A., GRING, H., & HARTUNG, A. (1986) Aldehyde emissions from passenger cars. Staub-Reinhalt. Luft, **46**: 136-139.

LIJINSKY, W. & ANDREWS, A.W. (1980) Mutagenicity of vinyl compounds in Salmonella typhimurium. Teratogen. Carcinogen. Mutagen., **1**: 259-267.

LIJINSKI, W. & REUBER, M.D. (1987) Chronic carcinogenesis studies of acrolein and related compounds. Toxicol. ind. Health, **3**: 337-345.

LIPARI, F. & SWARIN, S.J. (1982) Determination of formaldehyde and other aldehydes in automobile exhaust with an improved 2,4-dinitrophenylhydrazine method. J. Chromatogr., **247**: 297-306.

LIPARI, F., DASCH, J.M., & SCRUGGS, W.F. (1984) Aldehyde emissions from wood-burning fireplaces. Environ. Sci. Technol., **18**: 326-330.

LIU, Y. & TAI, H.-H. (1985) Inactivation of pulmonary NAD-dependent 15-hydroxyprostaglandin dehydrogenase by acrolein. Biochem. Pharmacol., **34**: 4275-4278.

LOQUET, C., TOUSSAINT, G., & LETALAER, J.Y. (1981) Studies on mutagenic constituents of apple brandy and various alcoholic beverages collected in Western France, a high incidence area for oesophageal cancer. Mutat. Res., **88**: 155-164.

LORZ, H.W., GLENN, S., WILLIAMS, R.H., KUNKEL, C.M., NORRIS, L.A., & LOPER, B.R. (1979) Effects of selected herbicides on Smolting Salmon, Corvallis, Oregon, USA Environmental Protection Agency, Environment Research Laboratory Corvallis, Office of Research and Development (Report EPA-600/3-79-071).

LOW, E.S., LOW, R.B., & GREEN, G.M. (1977) Correlated effects of cigarette smoke components on alveolar macrophage adenosine triphosphatase activity and phagocytosis. Am. Rev. respir. Dis., **115**: 963-970.

LUTZ, D., EDER, E., NEUDECKER, T., & HENSCHLER, D. (1982) Structure-mutagenicity relationship in α,β-unsaturated carbonylic compounds and their corresponding allylic alcohols. Mutat. Res., **93**: 305-315.

LYMAN, W.J., REEHL, W.F., & ROSENBLATT, D.H. (1982) Handbook of chemical property estimation methods, New York, McGraw-Hill Book Company.

LYON, J.P., JENKINS, L.J., JONES, R.A., COON, R.A., & SIEGEL, J. (1970) Repeated and continuous exposure of laboratory animals to acrolein. Toxicol. appl. Pharmacol., **17**: 726-732.

MACEK, K.J., LINDBERG, M.A., SAUTER, S., BUXTON, K.S., & COSTA, P.A. (1976) Toxicity of four pesticides to water fleas and fathead minnows, Duluth, Minnesota, US Environmental Protection Agency, Environmental Research Laboratory, Office of Research and Development, (Ecological Research Series EPA-600/3-76-099).

MCNULTY, M.J., HECK, H.D'A., & CASANOVA-SCHMITZ, M. (1984) Depletion of glutathione in rat respiratory mucosa by inhaled acrolein. Fed. Proc., **43**: 575 (abstract).

MAGIN, D.F. (1980) Gas chromatography of simple monocarbonyls in cigarette whole smoke as the benzyloxime derivatives. J. Chromatogr., **202**: 255-261.

MALDOTTI, A., CHIORBOLI, C., BIGNOZZI, C.A., BARTOCCI, C., & CARASSITI, V. (1980) Photooxidation of 1,3-butadiene containing systems: rate constant determination for the reaction of acrolein with OH radicals. Int. J. chem. Kinet., **12**: 905-913.

MANITA, M.D. & GOLDBERG, E.K. (1970) [Spectrophotometric analysis of airborne acrolein using the semithiocarbazide reagent.] Gig. i Sanit., **35**(5): 63-65 (in Russian).

MANNING, D.L., MASKARINEC, M.P., JENKINS, R.A., & MARSHALL, A.H. (1983) High performance liquid chromatographic determination of selected gas phase carbonyl in tobacco smoke. J. Assoc. Off. Anal. Chem., 66: 8-12.

MARANO, F. & DEMESTERE, M. (1976) Ultrastructural autoradiographic study of the intracellular fixation of ^{3}H-acrolein. Experientia (Basel), 32: 501-503.

MARANO, F. & PUISEUX-DAO, S. (1982) Acrolein and cell cycle. Toxicol. Lett., 14: 143-149.

MARINELLO, A.J., GURTOO, H.L., STRUCK, R.F., & PAUL, B. (1978) Denaturation of cytochrome P-450 by cyclophosphamide metabolites. Biochem. Biophys. Res. Commun., 83: 1347-1353.

MARINELLO, A.J., BERRIGAN, M.J., STRUCK, R.F., GUENGERICH, F.P., & GURTOO, H.L. (1981) Inhibition of NADPH-cytochrome P450 reductase by cyclophosphamide and its metabolites. Biochem. biophys. Res. Commun., 99: 399-406.

MARINELLO, A.J., BANSAL, S.K., PAUL, B., KOSER, P.L., LOVE, J., STRUCK, R.F., & GURTOO, H.L. (1984) Metabolism and binding of cyclophosphamide and its metabolite acrolein to rat hepatic microsomal cytochrome P-450. Cancer Res., 44: 4615-4621.

MARNETT, L.J., HURD, H.K., HOLLSTEIN, M.C., LEVIN, D.E., ESTERBAUER, H., & AMES, B.N. (1985) Naturally occurring carbonyl compounds are mutagens in Salmonella tester strain TA 104. Mutat. Res., 148: 25-34.

MASARU, N., SYOZO, F., & SABURO, K. (1976) Effects of exposure to various injurious gases on germination of lily pollen. Environ. Pollut., 11: 181-187.

MASEK, V. (1972) [Aldehydes in the air at working places in coal and pitch coking plants.] Staub-Reinhalt. Luft, 32: 335-336 (in German).

MASLOWSKA, J. & BAZYLAK, G. (1985) Thermofractographic determination of monocarbonyl compounds in animal waste fats used as feed fat. Anim. Feed Sci. Technol., 13: 227-236.

METTIER, S.R., BOYER, H.K., HINE, C.H., & MCEWEN, W.K. (1960) A study of the effects of air pollutants on the eye. Am. Med. Assoc. Arch. ind. Health, 21: 13-18.

MILLS, D.E., BAUGH, W.D., & CONNER, H.A. (1954) Studies on the formation of acrolein in distillery mashes. Appl. Microbiol., 2: 9-13.

MIRKES, P.E., GREENAWAY, J.C., ROGERS, J.G., & BRUNDRETT, R.B. (1984) Role of acrolein in cyclophosphamide teratogenicity in rat embryos *in vitro*. Toxicol. appl. Pharmacol., 72: 281-291.

MIYAMOTO, Y. (1986) Eye and respiratory irritants in jet engine exhaust. Aviat. Space environ. Med., 57: 1104-1108.

MORIKAWA, T. (1976) Acrolein, formaldehyde, and volatile fatty acids from smoldering combustion. J. Combust. Toxicol., 3: 135-150.

MORIKAWA, T. & YANAI, E. (1986) Toxic gases evolution from air-controlled fires in a semi-full scale room. J. Fire Sci., 4: 299-314.

MOULE, Y. & FRAYSSINET, C. (1971) Effects of acrolein on transcription *in vitro*. Fed. Eur. Biochem. Soc. Lett., 16: 216-218.

MULDERS, E.J. & DHONT, J.H. (1972) The odour of white bread. III. Identification of volatile carbony compounds and fatty acids. Z. Lebensm. Unters. Forsch., 150: 228-232.

MUNSCH, N. & FRAYSSINET, C. (1971) Action de l'acroléine sur les syntheses d'acides nucléiques *in vivo*. Biochimie, 53: 243-248.

MUNSCH, N., DE RECONDO, A.-M., & FRAYSSINET, C. (1973) Effects of acrolein on DNA synthesis *in vitro*. Fed. Eur. Biochem. Soc. Lett., 30: 286-289.

MUNSCH, N., MARANO, F., & FRAYSSINET, C. (1974a) Incorporation d'acroleine ^{3}H dans le foie du rat et chez *Dunaliella bioculata*. Biochimie, 56: 1433-1436.

MUNSCH, N., DE RECONDO, A.-M., & FRAYSSINET, C. (1974b) *In vitro* binding of ^{3}H-acrolein to regenerating rat liver DNA polymerase. Experientia, 30: 1234-1236.

MURPHY, S.D. (1965) Mechanism of the effect of acrolein on rat liver enzymes. Toxicol. appl. Pharmacol., 7: 833-843.

MURPHY, S.D. & PORTER, S. (1966) Effects of toxic chemicals on some adaptive liver enzymes, liver glycogen, and blood glucose in fasted rats. Biochem. Pharmacol., 15: 1665-1676.

MURPHY, S.D., KLINGSHIRN, D.A., & ULRICH, C.E. (1963) Respiratory response of guinea pigs during acrolein inhalation and its modification by drugs. J. Pharmacol. exp. Ther., 141: 79-83.

MURPHY, S.D., DAVIS, H.V., & ZARATZIAN, V.L. (1964) Biochemical effects in rats from irritating air contaminants. Toxicol. appl. Pharmacol., 6: 520-528.

NATUSCH, D.F.S. (1978) Potentially carcinogenic species emitted to the atmosphere by fossil-fueled power plants. Environ. Health Perspect., 22: 79-90.

NIELSEN, G.D., BAKBO, J.C., & HOLST, E. (1984) Sensory irritation and pulmonary irritation by airborne allyl acetate, allyl alcohol, and allyl ether compared to acrolein. Acta pharmacol. toxicol., 54: 292-298.

NISHIKAWA, H., HAYAKAWA, T., & SAKAI, T. (1986) Determination of micro amounts of acrolein in air by gas chromatography. J. Chromatogr., 370: 327-332.

NISHIKAWA, H., HAYAKAWA, T., & SAKAI, T. (1987a) Gas chromatographic determination of acrolein in rain water using bromination of *O*-methyloxime. Analyst, 112: 45-48.

NISHIKAWA, H., HAYAKAWA, T., & SAKAI, T. (1987b) Determination of acrolein and crotonaldehyde in automobile exhaust gas by gas chromatography with electron-capture detection. Analyst, 112: 859-862.

OBERDORFER, P.E. (1971) The determination of aldehydes in automobile exhaust gas. In: Vehicle emissions, Part III, Society of Automotive Engineers Prog. Tech., Vol. 14, pp. 32-42.

OHARA, T., SATO, T., SHIMUZU, N., PRESCHER, G., SCHWIND, H., & WEIBURG, O. (1987) Acrolein and methacrolein. In: Encyclopedia of chemical technology, Deerfield Beech, Florida, Ullmann Verlag Chemie.

O'LOUGHLIN, E.M. & BOWMER, K.H. (1975) Dilution and decay of aquatic herbicides in flowing channels. J. Hydrol., 26: 217-235.

OLSON, K.L. & SWARIN, S.J. (1985) Determination of aldehydes and ketones by derivatization and liquid chromatography-mass spectrometry. J. Chromatogr., 333: 337-347.

OSBORNE, A.D., PITTS, J.N., & DARLEY, E.F. (1962) On the stability of acrolein towards photooxidation in the near ultra-violet. Int. J. Air Water Pollut., 6: 1-3.

PATEL, J.M., WOOD, J.C., & LEIBMAN, K.C. (1980) The biotransformation of allyl alcohol and acrolein in rat liver and lung preparations. Drug Metab. Disposal, 8: 305-308.

PATEL, J.M., ORTIZ, E., KOLMSTETTER, C., & LEIBMAN, K.C. (1984) Selective inactivation of rat lung and liver microsomal NADPH-cytochrome c reductase by acrolein. Drug Metab. Disposal, 12: 460-463.

PEREZ, J.M., LIPARI, F., & SEIZINGER, D.E. (1984) Cooperative development of analytical methods for diesel emissions and particulates - solvent extractables, aldehydes and sulfate methods. In: Diesel exhaust emissions, Society of Automotive Engineers, pp. 95-114 (Special Publication No. 578).

PETTERSSON, B., CURVALL, M., & ENZELL, C.R. (1980) Effects of tobacco smoke compounds on the noradrenaline induced oxidative metabolism in isolated brown fat cells. Toxicology, 18: 1-15.

PFAFFLI, P. (1982) III. Industrial hygiene measurements. Scand. J Work Environ. Health, 8(suppl. 2): 27-43.

PHILIPPIN, C., GILGEN, A., & GRANDJEAN, E. (1970) Etude toxicologique et physiologique de l'acroléine chez la souris. Int. Arch. Arbeitsmed., 26: 281-305.

PILOTTI, A., ANCKER, K., ARRHENIUS, E., & ENZELL, C. (1975) Effects of tobacco and tobacco smoke constituents on cell multiplication *in vitro*. Toxicology, 5: 49-62.

PLOTNIKOVA, M.M. (1957) [Data on hygienic evaluation of acrolein as a pollution of the atmosphere.] Gig. i Sanit., 22(6): 10-15 (in Russian).

POSTEL, W. & ADAM, L. (1983) [Gas chromatographic characterization of raspberry brandy.] Dtsch. Lebensm. Rundschau, 79: 117-122 (in German).

POTTS, W.J., LEDERER, T.S., & QUAST, J.F. (1978) A study of the inhalation toxicity of smoke produced upon pyrolysis and combustion of polyethylene foams. Part I. Laboratory studies. J. Combust. Toxicol., 5: 408-433.

PRESSMAN, D. & LUCAS, H.J. (1942) Hydration of unsaturated compounds. XI. Acrolein and acrylic acid. J. Am. Chem. Soc., 64: 1953-1957.

PROTSENKO, G.A., TRUBILKO, V.I., & SAVCHENKOV, V.A. (1973) Working conditions when metals to which primer has been applied are welded evaluated from the health and hygiene aspect. Avt. Svarka, 2: 65-68.

RANDALL, T.L. & KNOPP, P.V. (1980) Detoxification of specific organic substances by wet oxidation. J. Water Pollut. Control Fed., 52: 2117-2130.

RAPOPORT, I.A. (1948) [Mutations under the influence of unsaturated aldehydes.] Dokl. Akad. Nauk. SSSR, 16: 713-715 (in Russian).

RATHKAMP, G., TSO, T.C., & HOFFMANN, D. (1973) Chemical studies on tobacco smoke. XX: Smoke analysis of cigarettes made from bright tobaccos differing in variety and stalk positions. Beitr. Tabakforsch., 7: 179-189.

RENZETTI, N.A. & BRYAN, R.J. (1961) Atmospheric sampling for aldehydes and eye irritation in Los Angeles smog. J. Air Pollut. Control Assoc., 11: 421-424, 427.

RICHTER, M. & ERFURTH, I. (1979) [On the gas chromatographic determination of acrolein in its original state in the main stream smoke of cigarettes.] Ber. Inst. Tabaksforsch. 26: 36-45 (in German).

RICKERT, W.S., ROBINSON, J.C., & YOUNG, J.C. (1980) Estmating the hazards of "less hazardous" cigarettes. I. Tar, nicotine, carbon monoxide, acrolein, hydrogen cyanide, and total aldehyde deliveries of Canadian cigarettes. J. Toxicol. environ. Health, 6: 351-365.

RIETZ, B. (1985) Determination of three aldehydes in the air of working environments. Anal. Lett., 18(A19): 2369-2379.

RIJSTENBIL, J.W. & VAN GALEN, G.C. (1981) Chemical control of mussel settlement in a cooling water system using acrolein. Environ, Pollut., A25: 187-195.

RIKANS, L.E. (1987) The oxidation of acrolein by rat liver aldehyde dehydrogenases. Relation to allyl alcohol hepatoxicity. Metab. Disposal, 15: 356-362.

ROSENTHALER, L. & VEGEZZI, G. (1955) [Acrolein in spirits.] Z. Lebensm. Unters. Forsch., 102: 117-123 (in German).

RYLANDER, R. (1973) Toxicity of cigarette smoke components: free lung cell response in acute exposures. Am. Rev. respir. Dis., 108: 1279-1282.

SAITO, T., TAKASHINA, T., YANAGISAWA, S., & SHIRAI, T. (1983) [Determination of trace low molecular weight aliphatic compounds in auto exhaust by gas chromatography with a glass capillary column.] Bunseki Kagaku, 32: 33-38 (in Japanese).

SAKATA, T., SMITH, R.A., GARLAND, E.M., & COHEN, S.M. (1989) Rat urinary bladder epithelial lesions induced by acrolein. J. environ. Pathol. Toxicol., 9: 159-170.

SALAMAN, M.H. & ROE, F.J.C. (1956) Further tests for tumour-initiating activity: N,N-di-(2-chloroethyl)-p-aminophenylbutyric acid (CB1348) as an initiator of skin tumour formation in the mouse. Br. J. Cancer, 10: 363-378.

SALEM, H. & CULLUMBINE, H. (1960) Inhalation toxicities of some aldehydes. Toxicol. appl. Pharmacol., 2: 183-187.

SCHAFER, E.W. (1972) The acute oral toxicity of 369 pesticidal, pharmaceutical and other chemicals to wild birds. Toxicol. appl. Pharmacol., 21: 315-330.

SCHIELKE, D.-J. (1987) [Gastrectomy following a rare caustic lesion.] Chirurg, 58: 50-52 (in German).

SCHMID, B.P., GOULDING, E., KITCHIN, K., & SANYAL, M.K. (1981) Assessment of the teratogenic potential of acrolein and cyclophosphamide in a rat embryo culture system. Toxicology, 22: 235-243.

SCHUCK, E.A. & RENZETTI, N.A. (1960) Eye irritants formed during photo-oxidation of hydrocarbons in the presence of oxides of nitrogen. J. Air Pollut. Control Assoc., 10: 389-392.

SCHUTTE, N.P. (1977) Hazard evaluation and technical assistance report No. TA 77-11: Xomed Company, Cincinnati, Ohio, Cincinnati, Ohio, USA, National Institute for Occupational Safety and Health (NIOSH-TR-TA-77-11, PB 278834).

SEIZINGER, D.E. & DIMITRIADES, B. (1972) Oxygenates in exhaust from simple hydrocarbon fuels. J. Air Pollut. Control Assoc., 22: 47-51.

SERTH, R.W., TIERNEY, D.R., & HUGHES, T.W. (1978) Source assessment: acrylic acid manufacture, Cincinnati, Ohio, US Environmental Protection Agency, Industrial Environmental Research Laboratory (Report EPA-600/2-78-004w).

SHAPIRO, R., SODUM, R.S., EVERETT, D.W., & KUNDU, S.K. (1986) Reactions of nucleosides with glyoxal and acrolein. In: The role of cyclic nucleic acid adducts in carcinogenesis and mutagenesis, Proceedings of a meeting organized by the IARC and co-sponsored by the US National Cancer Institute, and the Lawrence Berkely Laboratory at the University of California, Lyon, 17-19 September, Lyon, International Agency for Research on Cancer, pp. 165-173 (IARC Scientific Publications No. 70).

SHERWOOD, R.L., LEACH, C.L., HATOUM, N.S., & ARANYI, C. (1986) Effects of acrolein on macrophage functions in rats. Toxicol. Lett., 32: 41-49.

SHIMOMURA, M., YOSHIMATSU, F., & MATSUMOTO, F. (1971) [Fish odour of cooked horse mackerel.] Kaseigaku Zasshi, 2: 106-112 (in Japanese).

SIM, V.M. & PATTLE, R.E. (1957) Effect of possible smog irritants on human subjects. J. Am. Med. Assoc., 165: 1908-1913.

SINKUVENE, D. (1970) [Hygienic assessment of acrolein as an atmospheric pollutant.] Gig. i Sanit., 35(3): 6-10 (in Russian).

SKOG, E. (1950) A toxicological investigation of lower aliphatic aldehydes. I. Toxicity of formaldehyde, acetaldehyde, propionaldehyde and butyraldehyde, as well as of acrolein and crotonaldehyde. Acta pharmacol., 6: 299-318.

SLOTT, V.L. & HALES, B.F. (1985) Teratogenicity and embryolethality of acrolein and structurally related compounds in rats. Teratology, 32: 65-72.

SLOTT, V.L. & HALES, B.F. (1986) The embryolethality and teratogenicity of acrolein in cultured rat embryos. Teratology, 34: 155-163.

SLOTT, V.L. & HALES, B.F. (1987a) Enhancement of the embryotoxicity of acrolein, but not phosphoramide mustard, by glutathione depletion in rat embryos *in vitro*. Biochem. Pharmacol., **36**: 2019-2025.

SLOTT, V.L. & HALES, B.F. (1987b) Protection of rat embryos in culture against the embryotoxicity of acrolein using exogenous glutathione., Biochem. Pharmacol., **36**: 2087-2194.

SMITH, R.A., COHEN, S.M., & LAWSON, T.A. (1990) Acrolein mutagenicity in the V79 assay. Carcinogenesis, **11**: 497-498.

SMYTH, H.F., CARPENTER, C.P., & WEIL, C.S. (1951) Range-finding toxicity data: list IV. Arch. ind. Hyg. occup. Med., **4**: 119-122.

SMYTHE, R.J. & KARASEK, F.W. (1973) The analysis of diesel engine exhaust for low-molecular-weight carbonyl compounds. J. Chromatogr., **86**: 228-231.

SNYDER, J.M., FRANKEL, E.N., & SELKE, E. (1985) Capillary gas chromatographic analyses of headspace volatiles from vegetable oils. J. Am. Oil Chem. Soc., **6**: 1675-1679.

SPONHOLZ, W.-R. (1982) [Analysis and occurrence of aldehydes in wines.] Z. Lebensm. Unters. Forsch., **174**: 458-462 (in German).

SPRINCE, H., PARKER, C.M., & SMITH, G.G. (1979) Comparison of protection by L-ascorbic acid, L-cysteine, and adrenergic-blocking agents against acetaldehyde, acrolein, and formaldehyde toxicity: implications in smoking. Agents Actions, **9**: 407-414.

STACK, V.T. (1957) Toxicity of α,β-unsaturated carbonyl compounds to microorganisms. Ind. eng. Chem., **49**: 913-917.

STAHLMANN, R., BLUTH, U., & NEUBERT, D. (1985) Effects of the cyclophosphamide metabolite acrolein in mammalian limb bud cultures. Arch. Toxicol., **57**: 163-167.

STEINHAGEN, W.H. & BARROW, C.S. (1984) Sensory irritation structure-activity study of inhaled aldehydes in B6C3F1 and Swiss-Webster mice. Toxicol. appl. Pharmacol., **72**: 495-503.

STEPHENS, E.R., DARLEY, E.F., TAYLOR, O.C., & SCOTT, W.E. (1961) Photochemical reaction products in air pollution. Int. J. Air Water Pollut., **4**: 79-100.

SUBDEN, R.E., KRIZUS, A., & AKHTAR, M. (1986) Mutagen content of Canadian apple eau-de-vie. Can. Inst. Food Sci. Technol. J., **19**: 134-136.

SUZUKI, Y. & IMAI, S. (1982) Determination of traces of gaseous acrolein by collection on molecular sieves and fluorimetry with o-aminobiphenyl. Anal. Chim. Acta, **136**: 155-162.

SWARIN, S.J. & LIPARI, F. (1983) Determination of formaldehyde and other aldehydes by high performance liquid chromatography with fluorescence detection. J. liq. Chromatogr., **6**: 425-444.

SZOT, R.J. & MURPHY, S.D. (1971) Relationships between cyclic variations in adrenocortical secretory activity in rats and the adrenocortical response to toxic chemical stress. Environ. Res., 4: 530-538.

TABAK, H.H., QUAVE, S.A., MASHNI, C.E., & BARTH, E.F. (1981) Biodegradability studies with organic priority pollutant compounds. J. Water Pollut. Control Fed., 53: 1503-1517.

TAJIMA, M., KIDA, K., & FUJIMAKI, M. (1967) Effect of gamma irradiation on volatile compounds from cooked potato. Agric. biol. Chem., 31: 935-938.

TAKEUCHI, K. & IBUSUKI, T. (1986) Heterogeneous photochemical reactions of a propylene-nitrogen dioxide-metal oxide-dry air system. Atmos. Environ., 20: 1155-1160.

TEJADA, S.B. (1986) Evaluation of silica gel cartridges coated *in situ* with acidified 2,4-dinitrophenylhydrazine for sampling aldehydes and ketones in air. Int. J. environ. anal. Chem., 26: 167-185.

TESTA, A. & JOIGNY, C. (1972) Dosage par chromatographie en phase gazeuse de l'acroléine et d'autres composés α,β-insaturés de la phase gazeuse de la fumée de cigarette. Ann. Serv. Exploit. ind. Tab. Allumettes - Div. Etud. Equip., 10: 67-81.

TORAASON, M., LUKEN, M.E., BREITENSTEIN, M., KRUEGER, J.A., & BIAGINI, R.E. (1989) Comparative toxicity of allylamine and acrolein in cultured myocytes and fibroblasts from neonatal rat heart. Toxicology, 56: 107-117.

TREITMAN, R.D., BURGESS, W.A., & GOLD, A. (1980) Air contaminants encountered by firefighters. Am. Ind. Hyg. Assoc. J., 41: 796-802.

TURUK-PCHELINA, Z.F. (1960) [Acrolein releases into the air while cooking.] Gig. i Sanit., 25(5): 96-97 (in Russian).

UMANO, K. & SHIBAMOTO, T. (1987) Analysis of headspace volatiles from overheated beef fat. J. agric. food Chem., 35: 14-18.

UNRAU, G.O., FAROOQ, M., DAWOOD, I.K., MIGUEL, L.C., & DAZO, B.C. (1965) Field trials in Egypt with acrolein herbicide-molluscicide. World Health Organ. Bull., 32: 249-260.

US-NIOSH (1984) NIOSH manual of analytical methods, 3rd ed., Cincinnati, Ohio, National Institute for Occupational Safety and Health (DHHS (NIOSH) Publication No. 84-100. Method 2501).

VAN EICK, A.J. (1977) [The effect of acrolein in air on the eye blinking frequency of man and guinea pig], Rijswijk, The Netherlands, Technical and Physical Research, Medical Biological Laboratory, TNO-MBL, (Report No. A76/K/098) (in Dutch).

VAN OVERBEEK, J., HUGHES, W.J., & BLONDEAU, R. (1959) Acrolein for the control of water weeds and disease-carrying water snails. Science, 129: 335-336.

VEITH, G.D., MACEK, K.J., PETROCELLI, S.R., & CARROL, J. (1980) An evaluation of using partition coefficients and water solubility to estimate bioconcentration factors for organic chemicals in fish. Aquat. Toxicol.: 116-129.

VOLKOVA, Z.A. & BAGDINOV, Z.M. (1969) [Industrial hygiene problems in vulcanization processes of rubber production]. Gig. i Sanit., **34**: 33-40 (in Russian).

VOROB'EVA, A.I., VOLKOTRUB, L.P., FEOKTISTOVA, N.F., BOBIN, V.I., SHESTAKOVA, N.A., & USHAKOVA, N.S. (1982) [Characteristics of atmospheric pollution from enameled wire manufacturing plants.] Gig. i Sanit., **1982**(6): 66-67 (in Russian).

WARHOLM, M., HOLMBERG, B., & MALMFORS, T. (1984) The cytotoxicity of some organic solvents. Environ. Res., **7**: 183-192.

WATANABE, T. & AVIADO, D.M. (1974) Functional and biochemical effects on the lung following inhalation of cigarette smoke and constituents. II. Skatole, acrolein, and acetaldehyde. Toxicol. appl. Pharmacol. **30**: 201-209.

WEBER-TSCHOPP, A., FISCHER, T., & GRANDJEAN, E. (1976) [Objective and subjective physiological effects of passive smoking.] Int. Arch. occup. environ. Health, **37**: 277-288 (in German).

WEBER-TSCHOPP, A., FISCHER, T., GIERER, R., & GRANDJEAN, E. (1977) [Experimental irritation by acrolein in human beings.] Z. Arbeitswiss., **32**: 166-171 (in German).

WHITEHOUSE, M.W., BECK, F.W.J., DROGE, M.M., & STRUCK, R.F. (1974) Lymphocyte deactivation by (potential immunosuppressant) alkylating metabolites of cyclophosphamide. Agents Actions, **4**: 117-123.

WHO (1991) Health and Safety Guide 67: Acrolein, Geneva, World Health Organization.

WILMER, J.L., EREXSON, G.L., & KLIGERMAN, A.D. (1986) Attenuation of cytogenetic damage by 2-mercaptoethanesulphonate in cultured human lymphocytes exposed to cyclophosphamide and its reactive metabolites. Cancer Res., **46**: 203-210.

WILTON, D.C. (1976) Acrolein, an irreversible active-site-directed inhibitor of deoxyribose 5-phosphate aldolase? Biochem. J., **153**: 495-497.

WITZ, G., LAWRIE, N.J., AMORUSO, M.A., & GOLDSTEIN, B.D. (1987) Inhibition by reactive aldehydes of superoxide anion radical production from stimulated polymorphonuclear leukocytes and pulmonary alveolar macrophages. Biochem. Pharmacol., **36**: 721-726.

WRABETZ, E., PETER, G., & HOHORST, H.J. (1980) Does acrolein contribute to the cytotoxicity of cyclophosphamide? J. Cancer Res., **98**: 119-126.

ZIMMERING, S., MASON, J.M., VALENCIA, R., & WOODRUFF, R. (1985) Chemical mutagenesis testing in *Drosophila*. II. Results of 20 coded compounds tested for the National Toxicology Program. Environ. Mutagen., **7**: 87-100.

ZITTING, A. & HEINONEN, T. (1980) Decrease of reduced glutathione in isolated rat hepatocytes caused by acrolein, acrylonitril, and the thermal degradation products of styrene copolymers. Toxicology, **17**: 333-341.

ZOLLNER, H. (1973) Inhibition of some mitochondrial functions by acrolein and methylvinylketone. Biochem. Pharmacol., **22**: 1171-1178.

ZORIN, V.M. (1966) [Acrolein-induced air pollution.] Zdravookhr. Belorussii, **1966**(7): 43-44 (in Russian).

RESUME

L'acroléine est un liquide volatil extrêmement inflammable dont l'odeur, âcre et suffocante, est très désagréable. C'est un composé très réactif.

En 1975, on estime que la production mondiale d'acroléine en tant que telle était de 59 000 tonnes. On en produit et consomme encore davantage comme intermédiaire pour la synthèse de l'acide acrylique et de ses esters.

On dispose d'un certain nombre de méthodes d'analyse pour la recherche et le dosage de l'acroléine dans divers milieux. On a fait état de limites inférieures de détection de l'ordre de 0,1 $\mu g/m^3$ dans l'air (chromatographie en phase gazeuse/spectrométrie de masse), de 0,1 $\mu g/l$ dans l'eau (chromatographie liquide à haute pression), de 2,8 $\mu g/litre$ dans les milieux biologiques (fluorimétrie), de 590 $\mu g/kg$ dans le poisson (chromatographie en phase gazeuse/spectrométrie de masse) et de 1,4 $\mu g/m^3$ dans les gaz d'échappement (chromatographie liquide à haute pression).

On a trouvé de l'acroléine dans certains produits d'origine végétale et animale et notamment dans des denrées alimentaires et des boissons. L'acroléine est utilisée principalement comme intermédiaire en synthèse organique, mais également comme produit biocide en milieu aquatique.

Des émissions d'acroléine peuvent se produire sur les lieux de production ou d'utilisation. Elles peuvent être importantes dans l'air à la suite de la combustion ou de la pyrolyse incomplète de produits organiques tels que combustibles, polymères de synthèse, dans certains aliments et le tabac. L'acroléine peut représenter jusqu'à 3-10 % des aldéhydes totaux présents dans les gaz d'échappement des véhicules à moteur. La consommation d'une cigarette fournit de 3 à 228 μg d'acroléine. L'acroléine est un produit d'oxydation photochimique de certains polluants organiques de l'atmosphère.

La population générale est essentiellement exposée par l'intermédiaire de l'air. Une exposition peut également se produire par voie orale par suite de la consommation de boissons alcoolisées ou de denrées alimentaires chauffées.

On a mesuré dans l'air des villes des concentrations moyennes d'acroléine atteignant environ 15 $\mu g/m^3$ avec des maxima allant jusqu'à 32 $\mu g/m^3$. A proximité d'installations industrielles et de pots d'échappement, des concentrations dix à cent fois plus élevées sont possibles. Les incendies peuvent donner naissance à

Résumé

des teneurs très élevées d'acroléine, de l'ordre du mg/m^3 d'air. A l'intérieur des habitations, on a observé que la consommation d'une cigarette par m^3 d'air dans un local en l'espace de 10 à 13 minutes produisait des concentrations en vapeurs d'acroléine de l'ordre de 450 à 840 µg/m^3. Sur les lieux de travail, on a signalé des teneurs dépassant 100 µg/m^3 dans des cas où l'on élevait la température de certains produits organiques, par exemple lors du chauffage ou du soudage de ces substances.

Dans l'atmosphère, l'acroléine est dégradée par réaction avec les radicaux hydroxyles. Sa durée de séjour dans l'atmosphère est de l'ordre d'une journée. Dans les eaux de surface, l'acroléine se dissipe en quelques jours. Elle est faiblement adsorbée aux particules du sol. On a fait état de dégradation aérobie et anaérobie, encore que la toxicité du composé pour les micro-organismes puisse faire obstacle à sa biodégradation. Compte tenu des propriétés physiques et chimiques de l'acroléine, il ne semble pas que cette substance ait une tendance à la bioaccumulation.

L'acroléine est extrêmement toxique pour les organismes aquatiques. Pour les bactéries, les algues, les crustacés et les poissons, sa toxicité aiguë, estimée d'après les valeurs de la CE$_{50}$ et de la CL$_{50}$, se situe entre 0,02 et 2,5 mg/litre, les bactéries étant l'espèce la plus sensible. Pour le poisson, on a fixé à 0,0114 mg/litre la dose sans effet nocif observable à 60 jours. L'acroléine détruit efficacement les végétaux aquatiques à des doses comprises entre 4 et 26 mg/litre.h. A partir de 15 mg/litre, on observe des effets nocifs sur les cultures irriguées au moyen d'eau traitée à l'acroléine.

Chez l'homme et l'animal, l'acroléine reste confinée sur son site d'exposition en raison de sa réactivité et les observations pathologiques sont également limitées à ce site. Chez des chiens exposés à des doses de 400 à 600 mg/m^3, on a observé un taux de rétention de 80 à 85 % au niveau des voies respiratoires. L'acroléine réagit directement sur les groupements sulfhydryles protéiques et non protéiques ainsi que sur les amines primaires et secondaires. Elle peut également être métabolisée en acide mercapturique, en acide acrylique, en glycidaldéhyde ou en glycéraldéhyde. Les trois derniers métabolites n'ont été observés qu'*in vitro*.

L'acroléine est un agent cytotoxique. Sa cytotoxicité s'observe *in vitro* dès 0,1 mg/litre. Elle est extrêmement toxique pour les animaux de laboratoire et l'homme, à la suite d'une seule exposition quelle qu'en soit la voie. Sa vapeur est irritante pour l'oeil et les muqueuses respiratoires. Le liquide est corrosif et on a constaté qu'en solution éthanolique le seuil d'apparition d'une dermatite d'irritation était de 0,1%. L'expérimentation sur des volontaires humains exposés à des vapeurs d'acroléine a permis de fixer à 0,13 mg/m^3 la dose la plus faible produisant des effets nocifs observables; à cette dose, une irritation des yeux se produit en l'espace de cinq minutes. En outre, les effets au niveau des voies respiratoires deviennent évidents à partir de 0,7 mg/m^3. Une seule exposition à des doses plus élevées entraîne une dégénérescence de l'épithélium respiratoire, des séquelles inflammatoires et une perturbation de la fonction respiratoire.

On a étudié sur des rats, des chiens, des cobayes et des singes les effets toxicologiques de l'inhalation continue d'acroléine à des concentrations de 0,5 à 4,1 mg/m^3. Des effets histopathologiques et des effets sur la fonction respiratoire ont été observés chez les animaux exposés à des teneurs supérieures ou égales à 0,5 mg/m^3 pendant 90 jours.

On a étudié sur divers animaux de laboratoire les effets toxicologiques d'expositions répétées par la voie respiratoire à des vapeurs d'acroléine, à des concentrations allant de 0,39 mg/m^3 à 11,2 mg/m^3. La durée de l'exposition allait de cinq jours à 52 semaines. En général, on a fait état chez la plupart des espèces exposées huit heures par jour à des concentrations de 1,6 mg/m^3 ou davantage, d'une réduction du gain de poids, d'une diminution de la fonction respiratoire et de modifications pathologiques au niveau du nez, des voies respiratoires supérieures et des poumons. Parmi les modifications anatomopathologiques figuraient une inflammation, une métaplasie et une hyperplasie des voies respiratoires. On a observé une mortalité importante après expositions répétées à des vapeurs d'acroléine à des concentrations dépassant 9,07 mg/m^3. Chez l'animal d'expérience, on a montré que l'acroléine provoquait une déplétion du glutathion tissulaire *in vivo* et une inhibition des enzymes *in vitro* par réaction sur les groupements sulfhydryles au niveau des sites actifs. Il existe quelques données selon lesquelles l'acroléine est susceptible d'amoindrir les défenses pulmonaires de l'hôte chez la souris et le rat.

L'acroléine peut produire des effets tératogènes et embryotoxiques lorsqu'on l'introduit directement dans l'amnios. Toutefois, l'absence d'effets chez des lapins à qui elle avait été injectée par voie intraveineuse à la dose de 3 mg/kg incite à penser que l'exposition de l'homme à l'acroléine ne devrait pas avoir d'effet nocif sur le développement de l'embryon.

Résumé

On a montré que l'acroléine interagissait avec les acides nucléiques *in vitro* et en inhibait la synthèse tant *in vitro* qu'*in vivo*. Sans avoir besoin d'être activée, elle produit des mutations géniques chez les bactéries et les champignons et induit des échanges entre chromatides soeurs dans les cellules mammaliennes. Dans tous les cas, ces effets se sont produits dans un intervalle de dose extrêmement limité qui était fonction de la réactivité, de la volatilité et de la cytotoxicité de l'acroléine. Une épreuve de mutation létale dominante chez la souris a donné des résultats négatifs. Les données disponibles montrent que l'acroléine est faiblement mutagène pour certains champignons et bactéries et certaines cultures de cellules mammaliennes.

Des hamsters ont été exposés pendant 52 semaines à des vapeurs d'acroléine à la dose de 9,2 mg/m^3, 7 heures par jour et 5 jours par semaine, puis ont été placés en observation pendant les 29 semaines suivantes; aucune tumeur n'a été observée. En exposant ces hamsters dans les mêmes conditions à des vapeurs d'acroléine et pendant la même durée avec, en outre, des doses intra-trachéennes hebdomadaires de benzo[a]pyrène ou des doses sous-cutanées une fois toutes les trois semaines de diéthylnitrosamine, on n'a pas non plus observé d'effets co-cancérogènes bien nets attribuables à l'acroléine. Des rats exposés par voie orale à de l'acroléine dans leur eau de boisson à des doses comprises entre 5 et 50 mg/kg par kg de poids corporel (quotidiennement, cinq jours par semaine pendant 100 à 124 semaines) n'ont pas présenté de tumeur. En raison du caractère limité de toutes ces épreuves, on estime que les données qui permettraient d'évaluer la cancérogénicité de l'acroléine chez l'animal d'expérience sont encore insuffisantes. De ce fait, il est impossible pour l'instant d'évaluer la cancérogénicité de l'acroléine pour l'homme.

Les différents seuils de concentration auxquels apparaissent les différents effets de l'acroléine sont les suivants : perception d'une odeur, 0,007 mg/m^3, irritation oculaire, 0,3 mg/m^3, irritation du nez et clignement des yeux, 0,03 mg/m^3, réduction de la fréquence respiratoire, 0,7 mg/m^3. Comme la concentration de l'acroléine dépasse rarement 0,03 mg/m^3 dans l'air des villes, elle n'est pas susceptible de constituer une nuisance dans les circonstances normales.

Du fait de sa forte toxicité pour les organismes aquatiques, l'acroléine présente un danger pour la faune et la flore aquatique à proximité ou sur les sites de décharge de déchets industriels, en cas de déversements et là où l'on utilise ce produit comme biocide.

1. RESUMEN

La acroleína es un líquido volátil, sumamente inflamable, con un olor pungente, asfixiante y desagradable. Se trata de un compuesto muy reactivo.

La producción mundial de acroleína aislada se calculó en 59 000 toneladas en 1975. Se produce y consume una cantidad aún mayor de acroleína como intermediaria en la síntesis de ácido acrílico y sus ésteres.

Se dispone de métodos analíticos para determinar la acroleína presente en diversos medios. Los límites mínimos de detección que se han comunicado son 0,1 $\mu g/m^3$ de aire (cromatografía gaseosa/spectrometría de masas), 0,1 μg/litro de agua (cromatografía líquida a alta presión), 2,8 μg/litro de medio biológico (fluorimetría), 590 μg/kg en peces (cromatografía gaseosa/espectrometría de masas), y 1,4 $\mu g/m^3$ de gases de escape (cromatografía líquida a alta presión).

La acroleína se ha detectado en algunos vegetales y animales, inclusive en alimentos y bebidas. La sustancia se usa principalmente como intermediaria en la síntesis química aunque también como biocida acuático.

Pueden producirse emisiones de acroleína en sus lugares de producción o de uso. Las emisiones importantes a la atmósfera se deben a la combustión incompleta o la pirólisis de materiales orgánicos como ser combustibles, polímeros sintéticos, alimentos y tabaco. La acroleína puede representar el 3-10% de los aldehídos totales presentes en los escapes de automóviles. El humo de un cigarrillo libera 3-228 μg de acroleína. La acroleína es uno de los productos de la oxidación fotoquímica de ciertos contaminantes orgánicos de la atmósfera.

La exposición de la población general se produce principalmente por el aire. La exposición por vía oral puede producirse por el consumo de bebidas alcohólicas o alimentos calentados.

En la atmósfera urbana se han medido niveles promedio de acroleína de hasta unos 15 $\mu g/m^3$ y niveles máximos de hasta 32 $\mu g/m^3$. En las cercanías de las industrias y junto a los caños de escape pueden registrarse niveles entre 10 y 100 veces superiores. Como resultado de incendios pueden hallarse niveles sumamente elevados en el aire, del orden de mg/m^3. En el aire cerrado de interiores, el consumo de un cigarrillo por m^3 de volumen de la habitación produjo en 10-13 minutos concentraciones de vapor de acroleína de 450-840 $\mu g/m^3$. En el medio ambiente laboral se han detectado niveles de más de 1000 $\mu g/m^3$ en situaciones que entrañaban aumento de temperatura de materiales orgánicos, por ejemplo durante la soldadura o el calentamiento.

La acroleína se degrada en la atmósfera por reacción con radicales hidroxilo. El tiempo de persistencia en la atmósfera es de aproximadamente un día. En aguas de superficie, la acroleína se disipa en pocos días. Tiene un bajo potencial de adsorción en el suelo. Se ha observado su degradación en condiciones aerobias y anaerobias, si bien la toxicidad del compuesto para los microorganismos puede impedir la biodegradación. En vista de sus propiedades físicas y químicas, es improbable que se produzca bioacumulación de acroleína.

La acroleína es sumamente tóxica para los organismos acuáticos. Los valores de la CE_{50} y la CL_{50} correspondientes a bacterias, algas, crustáceos y peces se encuentran entre 0,02 y 2,5 mg/litro, siendo las bacterias los organismos más sensibles. En peces se ha determinado que el nivel sin observación de efectos adversos (NOAEL) a 60 días es de 0,0114 mg/litro. Se ha conseguido combatir eficazmente los vegetales acuáticos con dosis de acroleína comprendidas entre 4 y 26 mg/litro.h. Se han observado efectos adversos en cultivos que crecen en suelos irrigados con agua tratada con acroleína en concentraciones de 15 mg/litro o más.

En el animal y en el ser humano la reactividad de la acroleína limita efectivamente la sustancia al lugar de exposición; los hallazgos patológicos se limitan asimismo a esos lugares. En el tracto respiratorio de perros expuestos a 400-600 mg/m^3 se encontró una retención del 80-85% de acroleína. La acroleína reacciona directamente con los grupos sulfhidrilo contenidos en radicales proteicos o no proteicos y con aminas primarias y secundarias. También puede ser metabolizado a ácidos mercaptúricos, ácido acrílico, glicidaldehído o gliceraldehído. Estos tres últimos metabolitos sólo se han encontrado *in vitro*.

La acroleína es un agente citotóxico. Se ha observado citotoxicidad *in vitro* con niveles de solamente 0,1 mg/litro. La sustancia es sumamente tóxica para los animales de experimentación y el ser humano tras una exposición única por diferentes vías. El vapor es irritante para los ojos y el tracto respiratorio. En estado líquido es corrosiva. Con respecto a la dermatitis irritante, se encontró que el NOAEL de la acroleína etanólica era de 0,1%. Los experimentos con voluntarios humanos expuestos a vapores de acroleína mostraron un nivel mínimo de observación de efectos (LOAEL) de 0,13 mg/m^3, dosis con la que los ojos pueden irritarse al cabo de cinco minutos. Además, se observan efectos en el tracto respiratorio a partir de 0,7 mg/m^3. Con exposiciones aisladas a niveles más altos, aparecen: degeneración del epitelio respiratorio, secuelas inflamatorias y trastorno de la función respiratoria.

Los efectos toxicológicos de la exposición por inhalación continua de concentraciones comprendidas entre 0,5 y 4,1 mg/m^3 se han estudiado en la rata, el perro, el cobayo y el mono. Se observaron efectos sobre la función respiratoria y trastornos histopatológicos cuando se expuso a los animales a niveles de acroleína de 0,5 mg/m^3 o más, durante 90 días.

Los efectos toxicológicos de la inhalación repetida de vapores de acroleína en concentraciones comprendidas entre 0,39 mg/m^3 y 11,2 mg/m^3 se han estudiado en diversos animales de laboratorio. Las duraciones de la exposición variaron entre 5 días y hasta 52 semanas. En general, se han documentado: reducción de la adquisición de peso corporal, disminución de la función pulmonar y cambios patológicos en la nariz, las vías aéreas superiores y los pulmones en la mayoría de las especies expuestas a concentraciones de 1,6 mg/m^3 o más, durante 8 h/día. Entre los cambios patológicos se observaron inflamación, metaplasia e hiperplasia del tracto respiratorio. Se ha observado un nivel significativo de mortalidad tras la exposición repetida a concentraciones de vapor de acroleína superiores a 9,07 mg/m^3. En animales de experimentación, se ha demostrado que la acroleína agota el glutatión tisular y que *in vitro* inhibe enzimas reaccionando con los grupos sulfhidrilo de los sitios activos. Hay limitada evidencia de que la acroleína pueda deprimir las defensas pulmonares en el ratón y la rata.

La acroleína puede inducir efectos teratogénicos y embriotóxicos si se administra directamente en el amnios. No obstante, el hecho de que no se observaran efectos en ratones a los que se inyectó 3 mg/kg por vía intravenosa sugiere que la exposición humana a la acroleína tiene pocas probabilidades de afectar al embrión en desarrollo.

Se ha demostrado que la acroleína interacciona con los ácidos nucleicos *in vitro* y que inhibe su síntesis tanto *in vitro* como *in vivo*. Sin activación, indujo mutaciones génicas en bacterias y hongos y provocó intercambios de cromátidas hermanas en células de mamíferos. En todos los casos esos efectos se produjeron en un margen muy reducido de concentraciones, limitado por la reactividad, la volatilidad y la citotoxicidad de la acroleína. Un ensayo de letalidad dominante en ratones dio resultado negativo. Los datos disponibles muestran que la acroleína es un mutágeno débil para ciertas bacterias, hongos y cultivo celular de mamífero.

No se encontraron tumores en hámsters expuestos durante 52 semanas a vapores de acroleína con una concentración de 9,2 mg/m^3 durante 7 h/día, 5 días a la semana, y observados durante 29 semanas más. Cuando se expusieron hámsters a vapores de acroleína en las mismas condiciones durante 52 semanas y, además, a dosis intratraqueales de benzo[a]pireno semanalmente o a dosis subcutáneas de dietilnitrosamina una vez cada tres semanas, no se observó una acción cocarcinogénica clara de la acroleína. La exposición de ratas por vía oral a la acroleína en el agua de bebida, en dosis comprendidas entre 5 y 50 mg/kg de peso corporal al día (5 días/semana durante 104-124 semanas) no indujo tumores. Dado el carácter limitado de todos esos ensayos, se considera que no se dispone de datos suficientes para determinar la carcinogenicidad de la acroleína en los animales de experimentación. En consecuencia, se considera asimismo imposible evaluar la carcinogenicidad de la acroleína para el ser humano.

Los umbrales de acroleína que causan irritación y efectos en la salud son 0,07 mg/m^3 en el caso de la percepción del olor, 0,13 mg/m^3 en la irritación ocular, 0,3 mg/m^3 en la irritación nasal y el parpadeo, y 0,7 mg/m^3 en la disminución del ritmo respiratorio. Puesto que el nivel de acroleína raras veces supera los 0,03 mg/m^3 en el aire urbano, es poco probable que alcance niveles molestos o nocivos en circunstancias normales.

En vista de la elevada toxicidad de la acroleína para los organismos acuáticos, la sustancia representa un riesgo para la vida acuática en las proximidades de las zonas donde se producen vertidos y escapes industriales, y en los lugares donde se usa como biocida.

www.ingramcontent.com/pod-product-compliance
Ingram Content Group UK Ltd.
Pitfield, Milton Keynes, MK11 3LW, UK
UKHW021309180426
11947UKWH00015B/1122